Acknowledgments

Thanks and bounteous buckets of gratitude to:

The amazing and wonderful friends who rallied around my family and me with love, energy, and enough power to run a major corporation;

Lucy Childs, who shepherded me through much editing and rewriting;

Mary Price, for her diligent first read of the manuscript;

Susan and Terry Whittaker, of Viewpoint Books (Columbus, IN), for their encouragement;

Liz Nolan-Greven, for learning how to change the dressing on my port, among a zillion other things!

The Unitarian Universalist Congregation of Columbus, Indiana for constant love and support;

All the nurses who took care of me, and continue to care for people with their unceasing commitment and love. (There were a few special ones and you know who you are—I love you);

Dr. Larry Cripe and Dr. Robert Nelson, both of whom saved my life and also became my friends;

Indiana University Medical Center, where healing is an art and a mission, for all the love and respect, from the doctors and nurses to technicians and housekeepers;

Indiana Repertory Theatre for being an artistic home and a place of love and support, from top to bottom;

My brothers and sisters and nieces and nephews and their children, for everything they did (and continue to do) for me;

Hannah Kolodjieski, whose bravery, generosity, and decency have spread far and wide, in life and after;

My sons, Lucas, Connor, and Jack, for being great people and for weathering the storm with grace and honesty and compassion. You are amazing young men.

And most of all to my husband, Tim, who saw it all, the ugliest and darkest parts of this journey and who, as many caregivers do, continued on with unimaginable reserves of strength and love, when often the most potent bit of help was taking out the trash or warming leftovers for the boys or making sure school and soccer and whatever else was on the schedule got done, those endless and tedious details, and still found ways to love me, reassure me, and take care of me. Our marriage is the rock of my life.

Special thanks goes to the "angels"
who made the second edition of this book possible.

A percentage of the proceeds from the sale of this book goes to benefit Be the Match®. To learn more about Be the Match® and its life-saving mission, visit BeTheMatch.org

My Beautiful Leukemia

Jan Lucas-Grimm

HB

HOOSIER BOOKS, INC.
INDIANAPOLIS, INDIANA

For information contact:

HOOSIER BOOKS, INC.
P.O. Box 17035
Indianapolis, Indiana 46217
www.hoosierbooksonline.com

To order additional copies or to contact the author, visit:
www.MyBeautifulLeukemia.com

ISBN 978-1-4507-1842-4

Interior book design by April Altman-Reynolds / Hoosier Books, Inc.

Book cover design by Angela Jackson Photography & Design
www.AngelaJacksonPhotography.com

Proudly printed and bound in the United States of America by
Printing Partners, Inc., Indianapolis, Indiana

Foreword
By Dr. Larry Cripe

She stands, shorn. She has no hair. She wears no clothes. The spaces between her ribs are deep; her arms and legs thin. Sometimes I worry that she is too thin, too frail to survive. Other times she seems distilled to the essence of resiliency; what remains is what is required. The double doors behind her are closed. There is no doubt, however, that she is on the inside. The doors are to keep her in, to keep her safe, for a while, from the world she longs to return to.

There is a picture window in the wall over her right shoulder. A brown path winds through a green featureless valley towards a blue cloudless horizon. To her left is a larger window—an observation window—that we cannot see through. On the other side of the window is her hospital room. She is in the protective environment hallway, alone.

At some point during her first prolonged hospital stay during which she received chemotherapy for her newly diagnoses leukemia, Jan Lucas-Grimm—with the colored pencils she had been given by a friend—drew the picture, now matted and framed, that hangs on my office wall.

It seems unlikely that Jan ever stood in the hallway in that condition. The imaginary nature of the scene is clear in the almost whimsical depiction of the sterile plastic bags of red blood cells and platelets floating above her, tethered to her by intravenous tubing that terminates in the catheter in her neck. But is this how she felt? Now that she has regained her voice and written her story we can ask this and many other questions.

Several years ago a professional cyclist named Lance Armstrong was diagnosed with and treated for metastatic testicular cancer. After recovering from the treatments, he went on to win the Tour de France several more times. He has written books about survival. There are many differences between acute leukemia and testicular cancer. In Jan's case conventional chemotherapy did not cure the disease and so an allogeneic stem cell transplant was required. There has not been a point when Jan could walk away. To this day, she receives care related to the transplant and the drugs necessary to allow her to survive the new bone marrow and immune system.

And yet she writes this book. And she titles it *My Beautiful Leukemia*. She shares the faith she had in the physicians and nurses who greeted her. She wonders at the trust she showed in subjecting herself to physical and radiographic examination, to punctures of skin and marrow, and to accept into her body the chemicals to kill the leukemia before the leukemia killed her. All to return to the path she was on before she was diagnosed with leukemia. And she leaves us in no doubt that to have faith in medicine, to trust the advice of physicians—comforted by the compassion and sure steady presence of her nurses—is to resign oneself to a suspended uncertainty. I was struck by the dead-on accuracy of her description of an allergic reaction to her first platelet transfusion. The event emblematic of the other life-threatening complications of life-sustaining treatments she continues to endure.

With a similarly accurate, dispassionate and characteristic voice we witness—because of her generosity—the challenges to marriage, family and friends. But her sense of amazement, of wonder, of tempered appreciation is vivid in each anecdote.

Lance Armstrong was cured of his metastatic testicular cancer and returned to win a major bike race a bunch of times. Jan's triumph, I find, is more satisfying because it is less tidy; because she is actively engaged in the nuts and bolts of survivorship—ongoing anxiety about relapse, financial implications, emotional turmoil. This book gives voice to those who do not return fully to the life before cancer. I think of Dr. Mannette in *A Tale of Two Cities* who was recalled to life. Jan was recalled to life, she is on the brown path in the valley, by medical technology. But there was a cost. Her triumph is to bear the cost and to feel compelled to share her story with all of us as it unfolds.

On Beginnings...

I would like to start at the beginning. I would like to be able to say: this is what happened and this is when it happened and this is how it started. But when does cancer begin? By the time most people know it's happening inside of them, it has already claimed its space and made a home for itself. The seeds of the disease are planted when the patient isn't looking, deep in the genes, on a cellular level, and in my case, deep in the marrow of my bones.

"Down to the marrow"—it's an expression that means to the very core, to the essence of a thing. So to have cancer in my bone marrow, in my blood, felt like the essence of me was diseased. How could this happen? When did it begin?

I grew up in a middle-class suburb of Detroit, the youngest of five. We all had big grassy yards lined with elm trees, we rode our bikes everywhere, we took the bus to school, and we ate what everyone else ate at that time: meatloaf, baked chicken, pork chops with overcooked vegetables and potatoes. We had french toast for breakfast, sandwiches and Campbell's soup for lunch. An occasional meal of burgers from the Big Boy or take-out Chinese was the extent of our fast food. We watched TV: "Bonanza", "My Three Sons", and "The Wonderful World of Disney" on Sunday nights. What about this life would plant the seeds for leukemia?

I grew up, went to college, traveled around a bit with friends, and landed in Chicago to begin my adult life. While working in about ten different jobs, then finally finding my niche working in the restaurant of the man I would eventually marry, I began to take acting classes.

At the ripe old age of twenty-nine, I began a new career as an actress. I worked in the theater and, as was common at that time in Chicago, I made commercials and industrial films and worked on the occasional movie being shot in town. I was vigilant about my health and my body; after all, as an actress on camera, how you look is everything.

So where did leukemia come from? I have pondered these questions until my head hurts. I have gone over and over my history and searched for reasons, coming up with only more perplexing questions. I have relived arguments I had with my father and remembered times when I went without sleep so I could party in college. I've recalled foods that I ate that had dyes or preservatives or pesticides in them, or chemicals I might have inhaled as I passed by a factory or a farmer spraying his fields. I went over tragedies I had weathered, times of sorrow and times of despair. I have experienced grief, deep grief; did this cause my genes to eventually trigger my DNA to send the devastating message to my cells, to become cancer cells? What went wrong? When did it begin inside of me?

I can't tell you when it started, but I can tell you when I found out that I had it. I was diagnosed with Acute Myeloid Leukemia on February 16, 2005. It came as a complete shock, although now, as I look back, there were red flags waving all over the place.

1

In the fall of 2004, I drove from my home in Indiana up to Lakeside Michigan, to the beach house of a dear friend of mine to celebrate her 50th birthday. This was a gathering of six artistic and creative women who are all food and wine connoisseurs and there was sure to be a feast. These were women with whom I had shared the majority of my adult life. In my twenties, I met my future husband, we started a restaurant and then we had a son, in that order. It was a heady time involving a group of idealistic and committed people for whom the restaurant was more than a job; it was a work of art and it was a family. These people formed the core of my community and my life as I launched into adulthood.

Twenty some years later, with a divorce behind me, a new life including my husband Tim, and my sons Lucas, Connor and Jackson, and more than one career under my belt, I was gathering again with these women who had always meant so much to me. We covered many topics that weekend. One of us was going through a difficult divorce, one was facing some serious health issues, one was struggling as a single mom, one was re-vamping her business. There was much advice dispensed over those two and a half days, during which I must have said, five or six times, "I am SO tired. I'm always so tired." The general consensus was that I was doing too much; it was time to get my boys working more around the house. "That's what you have those big, strong boys for, right?" "C'mon…put them to work, it's the best thing for them. That's how they learn to be men." Okay, we agreed, that's the ticket! I left for home rejuvenated and with a plan to get my boys doing chores. Chores!

But I was still tired.

In December, after much procrastination, I made myself go to my gynecologist to tend to a recurring irritation. The doctor examined me, prescribed some medication, and asked how I was doing. I told her I was tired, always tired, and that I had absolutely no energy. She suggested I might be depressed and might I like to try some Prozac? I said I didn't think I was depressed—I was TIRED, didn't she get that? She smiled kindly, as if she knew better than me, and quickly scribbled a prescription for Prozac, "just in case." *Whatever*, I thought. I took it home and tossed it in the wastebasket.

Christmas came, and with it a vicious cold, filling my sinuses and lungs with congestion and pain. I grew sicker and sicker until I could hardly move on New Years Eve. I ached everywhere and had a headache that originated at the base of my neck and could not be alleviated with aspirin or any over the counter painkiller, only ice packs. I never really recovered from that cold; I just got less sick. January passed with bitter cold and clouds, and life carried on with the many details of two sons in elementary school activities and the oldest son in college, but I was barely keeping up.

One morning, after our boys went into school, my friend Mary and I sat in my car drinking coffee. I told her I just could not "rev up" for anything. I was not just tired; I was deeply fatigued, in the very core of me. My youngest son Jack had complained that I was always too tired to shoot hoops with him or kick a soccer ball. He told me, frankly, that I was a dud. That was certainly a damning indictment, coming from a ten year old. Mary said maybe I had mono. She had had it before: mononucleosis. Wasn't that a disease teen-agers got from kissing and no sleep? I rolled my eyes at the thought. When she explained that the cure was to rest and stay home, I scoffed at the thought. "No way could I do that!" But after deliberating a few weeks, I finally made an appointment to get a blood test from a local clinic.

So on the morning of Feb. 16, 2005, I walked into the local health clinic to see a nurse practitioner and have blood tests. She introduced herself and asked me what seemed like endless questions regarding my health history before she would send me to the lab. I remember how perky she was; wearing lots of gold rings and necklaces and very red lipstick—I can see her in my mind's eye clearly. After hearing about my fatigue, my "utter exhaustion" as I was phrasing it, she said, "I think you might be depressed." And she left the room, returning with a one page survey. "Just answer those questions and we'll talk," she said. I answered them carefully; they were mostly about the quality of my life, about the interest I had in various aspects of it, about sexual interest, about my energy level. She took the completed form, scored it according to a formula, and said with surprise, "Hmmm, you're only mildly depressed." I had to smile and said, "Everyone I know is mildly depressed! Our kids are growing up, the price of gas is out of sight and cell phones are controlling our lives! Aren't YOU depressed?" I thought that was pretty funny, but she did not laugh. Instead, she suggested I just TRY Prozac. I said, "NO! I want to get well, and if I still seem depressed then we'll talk."

I headed for home, exhausted from the ordeal, and went to bed, to take what had become a routine: my afternoon nap. Around five o'clock, with the boys home from school and shooting baskets out back, I received a phone call. It was the nurse practitioner from the clinic wanting to talk to me. With the phone wedged between my chin and shoulder, I was telling my son Connor to set the table, looking up a recipe, and hearing this woman say in ominous tones that my white blood count was high. Very high. "Oh," I said brightly, "that's better than low, isn't it?" "Not exactly," she said. "The doctors here think…you might have…leukemia."

I think everyone remembers his or her moment of diagnosis. It is surreal. I honestly could not comprehend the words she was saying to me. I thought she might mean leprosy or lupus or lullabies or anything else that began with "L". Then I thought she was talking to the wrong person. I began to blabber. "No no no. Stop. I don't know what you mean. That can't be <u>me</u>. I don't understand. You don't understand. You must be wrong, you have the wrong person." Connor poked his head in the sunroom where I was on the phone. "Mom! What's wrong?" "It's the clinic," I whispered. "It's not cancer, is it?" he said worriedly. (What? How could he say that?) "Noooo," I whispered back. "Not cancer." Well, in my mind, I was right. She was talking about "leukemia", not cancer. Whatever the hell "leukemia" was.

Timing is everything, isn't it? My husband Tim, who is an actor as well as a composer and singer-songwriter, was up in Indianapolis rehearsing a play. He had composed music and was to be performing every night on stage in the Indiana Repertory Theatre's production of "Grapes of Wrath". That night was to be their very first audience. I had to call him. I reached the administrative offices of the theater and carefully said to the receptionist, "I need to speak to Tim Grimm. It's an emergency. Everybody's okay, but it is an emergency." She put me on hold for a few seconds, then came back on and said, in her languid Hoosier drawl, "All right now, they're going to get him in the theatre. See, the elevator isn't working, so someone's got to run all the way down there. You stay on now, Jan. Don't hang up. They told me to keep talking to you so you don't hang up." I had to smile. "I'm not going to hang up, Agnes, I need to speak to Tim." There was a pause. "Well, I don't know what in God's name to talk about!" "It's okay, we don't have to talk," I said. After a very long minute, Tim was on the phone, his ever-calm and stoic voice saying, "What's going on, honey?" I felt ridiculous saying it, I almost laughed. "Well, uh, the clinic called and they said I might have…*leukemia*." I could hardly get the word out of my mouth. So unreal, so completely bizarre to utter those words. Always unflappable, Tim said, "Okay, what are we supposed to do?" I told him I had been instructed to go up to Indiana University Medical Center in Indianapolis right away, about five minutes from where he was working. A doctor was expecting me. I had to make arrangements for the boys, but I would be up there as soon as possible. He said he'd meet me there.

This was the beginning of the mobilization of the troops, as we came to call them. These are my women friends in Columbus, Indiana, who went into action as soon as they heard the news. Mary took one boy, Suzanne took another, Carol agreed to drive me up to IU (Indiana University Medical Center), Liz began to make plans to see me the next day, and Cathy was making phone calls. All the way up I-65 to the hospital, Carol and I rode along in silence, repeating occasionally, "Well, we can't worry yet. We don't know exactly what it is." Right. Logic. Reason. These must prevail or we would both fall apart. We went up to floor 5-North and there, in the fluorescent light,

I saw a chilling sign: Hematology/Oncology. I just shook my head in wonder, sure that it was all a big mistake. I said I was there to see a Doctor Suva…something. They said, "Yes, Dr. Suvannasahnka, she's expecting you. Your room is at the end of the hall."

I was disarmed to see that a room already had my name on the door, and when I went in, I saw signs that said: "ISOLATION. MASK AND GLOVES REQUIRED" Wha-a-at? Did I have something catching? No, I was to find out, it was to protect <u>me</u> from other people's bugs. My immune system was apparently so compromised and ineffective, that I needed to be kept germ-free. This was all weird, and getting weirder by the minute.

I was sent back downstairs to register. My name was called and I went into a little cubicle to provide insurance information, phone and address, emergency contacts, and finally as it turned out, to get an explanation of a living will. Feeling slightly numbed by the dull gray walls of the cubicle and the tapping of the intake secretary's long painted nails on the keyboard, I was suddenly jolted into awareness by this question: A living will? Isn't that for people who are about to die? This couldn't really be germane to my situation and I emphatically said NO. I was so perturbed by that inquiry—how dare they ask me about such a thing when I might not even be sick?

Carol and I trudged back up to the fifth floor, where she would wait with me until Tim could be there. I remember noticing, as we returned to that room, how dim the lighting was, the colors seemed faded, the dusty pink and gray walls, the beige curtain around the bed, the gray curtain over the window that separated the room from the entryway. I shook my head as I looked around and almost laughed to find myself there; this couldn't be happening to me. Surely, there was a mistake.

An amazing bundle of energy and sarcastic humor burst into the room. This was one of the nurses, Debbie, who came in to take my vital signs, and start an IV. She explained that I was there because of a possible diagnosis of leukemia. "What IS leukemia?" I asked. She gave one of the best explanations of the disease I have ever heard. She said it is like 2,000 two-year-olds running around in your veins, not having a clue as to what they're supposed to do and not mature enough to do it. She also told me, as I was going to sleep, that she wouldn't see me until her next shift in five days. "Oh," I said, "I probably won't be here." She just looked at me. "Uh-huh," she said. Many days later, we would laugh about that. That was Day One of a thirty-day stay, my first of many hospital stays to come.

As I write about this now, after enduring so many tests and scopes and biopsies and tubes put in and tubes taken out, my take on the hospital experience is radically different than it was that first full day. Of course, that day would have to go down as one of the worst days in my life. I was unprepared for what I would need to do and what would have to be done to me to obtain a complete diagnosis. I had a chest x-ray, a fifteen-minute heart x-ray, a triple lumen inserted into the vein in my neck, and a bone marrow biopsy in my hip. I was so uninitiated in the ways of being a patient that I barely spoke during the whole day. I didn't speak up about the excruciating pain I was in, holding my head just so for insertion of the lumen. (This is a type of "port" for easy administration of medicines and chemo, as well as for easy withdrawal of daily blood samples, thus avoiding a need for multiple needle sticks into my arm. It proved to be an easier thing to live with than to insert.) I didn't call out that I was claustrophobic in the velcroed-in position for the heart picture, and I only whimpered a little during the biopsy.

Tim was able to be with me for the biopsy, at the beginning of that day. This procedure involves a little bit of numbing medication on one's hip area, and then a tool is inserted through the skin into the hip bone and into the actual marrow to get a core sample, much like a geologist going into rock. An inch long sample of the marrow is retrieved and then extruded from the pipette-like tool and taken to the lab. Having a needle inside the hipbone is a pain like no other, like something is in the basement of your bones, a place where it's not supposed to be. I had to keep my eyes riveted on Tim's face to keep my composure. After Tim left for work at the theatre, Liz took over and accompanied me to all the other tests. It was a grueling day and surreal, like a nightmare. The IU Cancer Center was undergoing a major rebuilding at that time, to become the amazing and beautiful Cancer Center that it is now, and so the facilities were crowded. Sometimes there was only a curtain to separate me from one or two other patients waiting to be examined, and often they were crying from grief or pain. Or vomiting. Or moaning. The hospital experience was thrown at me like a bucket of ice-cold water.

There was one thing that I kept in mind as I endured one variety of poking and prodding after another. The summer before, our son Connor had undergone surgery to remove part of his small intestine scarred from Crohn's disease. He had been in Riley Children's Hospital for five days (part of the same university campus as IU Med Center) and I stayed with him the entire time, on a narrow cot next to his bed. He had been through a battery of tests prior to the surgery. His bravery and his even-keeled attitude were astounding at the time, but even more so in hindsight for me, as I was going through tests that were not even as difficult as his had been. I remember one in particular, during which he was to have about 30 feet of tubing pushed down through his esophagus to his intestines with a small camera at the very end, to locate the exact place of the scar tissue. I was in the room with him during the prep while the doctor, a white-haired and extremely kind gentleman, was describing the process to me. His younger assistant had laid all the tubing on top of Connor's blanketed chest and Connor looked at it in horror and in a quivering voice, asked, "What is all of this??" The doctor quickly put the tubing down on the table next to him so Connor wouldn't have to look at what seemed like miles of clear tubing that were going to go inside of him. Connor, at that point, whispered to me, "I think you should go now, Mom. I think I can do this better by myself." What a hero. What a champ! I have often thought of his bravery throughout my whole adventure with leukemia and hospitals and tests, and it has given me courage to persevere.

My first days in the hospital were strange in their novelty; I obviously had never gone through anything like it before. It was actually interesting to experience such a new and different world; the sounds, the smells, the people. But in those early days, it had not sunk in how sick I was. The lovely Dr. Suvannasahnka explained that the diagnosis of acute myeloid leukemia (AML) was indeed confirmed, adding also that my heart looked very good so it would withstand the chemo. "Your heart is in great shape, both physically and poetically," she said with a knowing smile. "Your heart is very strong." I believed her. She explained that acute myeloid leukemia, also called acute myelogenous leukemia, is a quickly progressing disease in which too many immature blood-forming cells are found in the blood and bone marrow. She explained the course of treatment would be in two phases. The purpose of the first, "remission induction", is to kill the leukemia cells in the blood and marrow and achieve remission of the disease. The second phase, called "maintenance therapy", is designed to kill any remaining leukemia cells that may not be active but could begin to grow and cause a relapse.

I took in as much as I could understand in that overwhelming moment. Then I just wanted to get underway. When the nurse finally brought in the bag of chemo, I thought, "Here I go. I've heard about this. I've never imagined this would be me. But here it is and here I am. Bring it on."

I had said to Tim, during one of those chemo days, that I knew something amazing was going to come out of all this. I remember thinking that very thing on the night of my admission; even in my terrified state, I had a gut feeling that something very good would emerge from all of it. That had been my previous experience with other personal disasters: some amazing revelation or discovery or a very big growth step had come on the heels of such events. I told Tim that we had better get some good Art out of this; a couple of good songs and a poem or two, at least. I couldn't have predicted how much we would all actually gain from the illness, and also what we would lose.

2

During the first couple of days of chemo, I just felt tired and a little bit achy, not really sick. I kept wondering quietly to myself if it was really leukemia. I was giving myself over to the medical machine, the western way of doing things. I knew of others who had opted for "alternative" methods of healing, and truthfully, that sounded much nicer. I had always chosen alternative health care, such as homeopathy or acupuncture, or nutritional ways of dealing with sickness. But I couldn't bring myself to go down that path this time. I decided that cancer was bigger than anything I had come up against so far and that I would stay with the people who had devoted their lives to exploring, treating and curing this mysterious disease. It was a huge leap of faith. I am sure I was very influenced by the compassion and intelligence of all the nurses and doctors. If they had been rude and obnoxious or had appeared incompetent, my faith would have wavered.

At first, I was almost embarrassed to be the center of so much attention for what seemed like a mild case of the flu. My knowledge or experience of cancer was so minimal that I couldn't quite grasp what it meant to be a cancer patient. I thought I would be immediately in the throes of wrenching pain and distress. So when my friend Julia proposed a webpage for me to communicate about the illness, I balked. Who would want to go to a website about my leukemia? Boring! And depressing. And, as far as I could tell, pretty uninteresting. But Julia works at a hospital and knew about an organization designed for just this purpose: to communicate with the wider network of friends and family without having to talk about it everyday, or explain to each concerned individual how things were going. So, the "caringbridge" website was set up in my name, and friends began to write reports of my leukemia experience and the comings and goings of my treatment. My friend Janet came down from Chicago and actually took pictures, which went up on the website too. I could never have predicted or imagined the wide reach of this net over the next months, and how much support and love and encouragement it would offer to me. The home page of the website described its purpose:

> This website has been set up for Jan's friends and family to communicate about her illness and keep us all up to date on her progress without bothering her and Tim as they go through this hard time. Keep your positive vibes and prayers and meditations coming her way. They are sure to help in the healing.

And the first journal entries, written by my friends, read:

THURSDAY FEB. 17—Jan is going through tests to determine her diagnosis. It is believed she has leukemia. I am, like everyone else I'm sure, going to the web to find out what that means. Please post any news you may have of her because I may not know. -Julia

FRIDAY FEB. 18—Jan went through a lot of tests and they are waiting to get the results of everything before they administer the chemo. I understand that is so they give her exactly the right "cocktail" but she's impatient because she thinks the sooner she gets medication, the sooner she will get better. Makes sense to me. Chemo, cancer, leukemia—it's a new bunch of words to me and to Jan. It's all very new and scary and she needs her friends now like never before. Keep her in your prayers and meditations and whatevers… -Liz

FEB. 19, 2005—I talked to Tim's brother, Luke and his wife Esther, who had been with Jan today. They said she was in good spirits, but very tired. She also said Jan was having a hard time talking due to her cough, but they laughed a lot, no doubt because they were watching many episodes of Bonanza. Jan was also craving canned peaches or canned fruit cocktail (this from our health nut?) Okay, this is not a lot of news, but who needs more than Bonanza? -Maija

FEB. 21—Jan has pneumonia, it is definite. So more oxygen and breathing treatments, along with the antibiotics. Today is her birthday and while the chemo treatment and truckloads of pills are not the preferred birthday celebratory substances, as she said, "This is going to be a different kind of year." That's an understatement! -Julia

As I think now about those first days in the hospital, I am reminded that I was so naïve, well ignorant is a better word, about the ways of a hospital or about cancer and cancer treatment. I was so vastly unprepared for the situation that I just rolled along with it, birthdays notwithstanding. I don't know how I managed to pay such close attention to the doctors' explanations of things, or to the medications nurses would bring to me, or to any of the procedures I underwent. I was aware on some deep level that I had better pay attention. And I did. Now, even after years of treatment and medication (when I can hardly remember my own children's names or where I spent last Christmas) I can tell you every medication I am on, and have been on, for the last three and a half years. I don't know how it works, but I know that being "present" and involved has been crucial in my healing. There is no better judge of how a patient feels than the patient herself.

The pneumonia was a frightening thing to deal with. I had developed a deep fear that something other than leukemia would get me; that some complication or reaction to a medication or a side effect of my treatment would do me in rather than the leukemia itself. Pneumonia was one of many side trips that my illness would take, one of the many complexities of the medical journey that I was embarking on. Thus I felt I had to be ever vigilant in my own internal assessment, and always communicate it to the nurses. My biggest fear about pneumonia was that I would suffocate, or more accurately, drown in my own lung fluid. A pulmonary specialist came four times a day (or night) and hooked me up to a breathing machine filled with medicine to inhale, and her calm and confident ways reassured me tremendously. I had to quiet that fearful voice in my head, the one that was panicking on the inside, and focus on healing.

Visitors began to arrive. What an odd position to be in—to be the center of attention because I was sick, really sick. But I didn't even look sick, yet. I still had my long hair, I was relatively alert, and I was as energetic as I'd been for the last couple of weeks. Nothing had changed outwardly except there was this <u>diagnosis</u> hanging in the air. And there I was, in pajamas, sitting in the hospital. So I had to learn how to receive visitors. My first instinct was to entertain everyone. I felt so responsible for them being there; they had made such an effort to see me and what was there to see? I couldn't even provide the drama of real illness yet, no moaning, no raspy voice asking for ice chips, no juicy details. Of course, I would be utterly exhausted after the visitors left. It's hard work to keep up a conversation about…what? Do we talk about leukemia? Do we talk about mundane details of everyday life? Do we talk about death? Finally I realized I had to just allow for silence. I was not there to entertain, and as the weeks went by and I did become visibly sick, I learned how to do nothing. What I wanted most was to hear the visitors talk. I wanted to hear about life going on, about their kids and dogs and who they ran into in the grocery store. I wanted to hear who was reading what, who was talking to whom on the phone, how cold it was outside and how funny or exasperating or adorable their kids or spouses were.

It wasn't easy for the visitors either. They were shy to talk about the mundane in the presence of something as serious as leukemia. They waited for me to give them clues about what to do, and when I stopped doing that, there would be awkward silence. So we all had to learn together, realizing as the days went by, what was needed on both sides of the relationship.

Sometimes, people visited that I barely knew. They were "in the neighborhood", or they worked nearby and felt like stopping in. I don't know how that line of thinking works in a person's mind, but there was nothing harder than having to talk to people that I barely knew, let alone try to remember their names. It became apparent, as my hospital stay progressed, that some people had their own agendas for this illness; my illness was functioning in a certain way for them. I don't think this happened on a conscious level; rather it was part of the very human desire to be needed. But that desire can be taken to extremes when someone is seriously ill and I could feel my emotions become muddled when such energy entered the room. I was finally able to identify this predicament and realized that I needed to conserve all my energy for healing, not for worrying about other peoples' needs or wants from <u>their</u> experience of <u>my</u> illness. Yet this was a difficult concept to grasp, especially when I was so grateful for the efforts, energy and support from everyone. A couple of girlfriends decided that a schedule of visitors needed to be organized with one person serving as the "gatekeeper" so too many people wouldn't all come to the hospital at once. Kathleen, ever efficient and clear-headed, was the woman for the job. Again, we were all learning how to function in this new arena.

Even with a schedule to plan and coordinate visits, there were many hours of being alone. I found that I could not read; I didn't have the ability to concentrate. Television was positively moronic, and listening to music made me irritated. So I spent a lot of time just sitting, usually with my eyes closed. I found out that I didn't mind being alone, at least in the daytime, and would move from the bed to the big blue chair to the hard plastic desk chair, to get different perspectives on the room. I had so much to think about. It sounds funny to say, but I found that I liked myself, on the inside, in a way I had never known before. My mind wandered from the present to the past. Over the course of the next 30 days, I reviewed my life as I remembered things. As I walked through memories of childhood events, people from my past came drifting in and out of my consciousness. I saw the house I grew up in, my dog, my friends in the neighborhood. I remembered Michigan summer nights on our back porch and I remembered snowy February days, waiting for the bus. I saw my sisters and brothers and parents all in a collage of memory. I remembered how smart but emotionally volatile my father was, and I could see my mother presiding over the dinner table, so innately and beautifully kind but helpless to deal with the vagaries of his tumultuous moods. I remembered living in Chicago just out of college, moving to Los

Angeles, coming back to Indiana, being an artist, being a mother. All of this added up to a life, to the creation of Me, and now I had leukemia. Leukemia? It was hard, impossible even, to put that together with all the other strands of my life. Leukemia?

I wondered about the future. What would it be like to be a "survivor", a word I was hearing often. What would leukemia do to that person known as me, what would I become? While ruminating upon this, and a million other things, I liked to just sit and let my thoughts go where they would. Often a nurse would come in and be surprised to see me sitting with my eyes closed.

One time, a very well intended social worker came blustering in with lots of positive energy, and began to inquire, loudly, about my plans for my hair, or lack of it. "Have you read our brochures? Have you considered a wig? Have you seen the options for hats and turbans?" I had been so preoccupied and off in my own thoughts that her energy took me by surprise and I could only envision hats and wigs swirling around her head as she talked. No, I hadn't read the brochures, I hadn't read anything yet. In the drawer next to the bed, there was a huge pile of papers and pamphlets and brochures on cancer-this and cancer-that; you might want this but you might not want that and you have to pay for this and here's how you pay for that and it was all absolutely overwhelming. I began to giggle; out-of-control and giddy. I couldn't help it. I felt like I was in a movie, some oddball comedy with weird special effects. The room appeared to be spinning and it was all I could do to tell her that I didn't mind losing my hair and had no plans to get a wig. Not that I have anything against wigs, but I was more concerned with staying alive than worrying about my hair. For most of my life, my long blonde hair had pretty much defined my image, my "look", so it was kind of interesting not to care about it now, when I knew I was going to lose it. I giggled till I cried and the social worker gently backed out of the room with assurances to return at a "better" time. Poor thing.

I had some unlikely visitors. A gynecologist, a friend of a friend of a friend, popped in one time as I was asleep on the blue chair. He wanted to tell me he had just figured it out—he knew who I was related to, he'd seen my name on his chart and wasn't that GREAT?

And wasn't that WILD that he knew who I was and wasn't it a SMALL world? He didn't even notice he had awakened me and his voice got louder with each exclamation, and then poof! He was gone before I could utter a word.

Nighttime in the hospital was so different from daytime. As the light outside my window faded, so did my spirits. Dinner was a lonely event, and even if I did have visitors, I knew they eventually had to leave and I would be alone. Alone with my disease. I couldn't sleep. There was a constant, muffled noise from the hallway. A cart was wheeled by, or a bleep from my IV machine or from someone else's. There were sounds from other patient's televisions and voices over the hospital loudspeaker. When that voice would intone the end of visiting hours, I felt despair.

The room was never dark. There was a constant glow from the lights outside, leaking through the blinds. There was the constant glow from my IV machine. I tossed and turned, worried and confused, and often as I was finally falling asleep, a nurse would wake me to "take my vitals". At two in the morning, they wanted my blood pressure, temperature, heart rate, and blood oxygen level. It was like being in another country with different customs and language. I also wondered, as I grew sicker, if I might need a more clear thinking person in the room to help me understand a procedure or medication.

So after a couple of those scary nights, I told my friends that I would really like someone to spend the night with me if possible. I look back at this now and I can't believe that I had the absolute nerve to ask for this, and more astoundingly, that they actually did it! For 25 nights, I had one friend or another spend the night on "the blue chair". This was the big blue vinyl chair that folded back and out into a kind of sleeping chair/bed. (The word "bed" is putting it kindly; it wasn't even a cot!) It was <u>not</u> comfortable and it's hard to believe people actually spent the night on that thing. Not only that, but they had to wear a mask and gloves the whole time. I remember my first check-up in the Hematology Clinic after I had been discharged from that first stay, having to wear a mask and rubber gloves to protect myself from germs. The discomfort and claustrophobic feeling experienced then caused me to reflect on my friends spending a whole night like that, as well as their days with me. I marvel at their dedication and sacrifice and I can only hope I will be as generous if I'm ever asked to do the same. But there is much that I don't remember from that time because, as the chemo effects worsened, I had to rely on a morphine drip to ease my pain, and it wiped out most recollections of that time. But I do know now that the "Blue Chair People" did their share of helping me to the bathroom, helping me change pajamas, which I had to do once or twice a night due to night sweats, cleaning me up after vomiting and holding me when I cried. They helped me bathe and they rubbed my legs and feet with lotion. The Chicago women came down, my friend James came in from California, my sisters and one of my brothers came, our dear friends Rick and Laura came in from the west coast, and the nurses got to know my community of "peeps" as my oldest son called them.

Lucas was at Earlham College at the time, about an hour east of Indianapolis. The first thing he did on hearing the news of my diagnosis was to shave his head in solidarity with my baldness. He was dismayed to find that my hair had not yet fallen out when he first visited and he was as bald as a cue ball! He drove to the hospital every Friday after classes and stayed the evening with me. Often he would read from the website so I could hear what people had written. Some things made me laugh so hard that it would hurt my aching tummy and others made me fill up with gratitude and love. Every single entry over the long haul meant, and still means, a great deal to me.

I couldn't believe how the news spread. It was as if a large net had been cast out, bringing in a wide assortment of love and support while sending out information at the same time. This was the World Wide Web at its best. I heard from old friends I hadn't seen in years, old boyfriends, ex-in-laws, teachers of my boys, people who rented an apartment from me in Chicago and friends of friends who I didn't even know. Churches put me on their prayer list, from southern Indiana to New York City. Along with the e-mail, cards and letters started pouring in. One day a nurse came in with a big pile of letters and said that I had won the award for the most mail that day. I burst into tears. She was alarmed and said, "Sweetie, I'm sorry. What's wrong?" I said,

"Then why am I so sad?" It was starting to hit me deeply that I was sick, really sick, and that I might not make it and my children would be motherless and this could be the big "D". I felt as if a bottomless pit was opening inside of me. The specter of death and the image of my children growing up without me made me swoon with despair. What about their soccer games, and concerts and graduations? And even worse than that, in my dark and brooding view of the future, there was some *other* mother, some other woman who might take my place—aaach, no! Another life for my kids? I know one is supposed to be generous to their spouse when facing death, encourage them to go on living, "of course, you should remarry"—NO! I did not feel that way. In fact, in one hysterical weeping fit, I believe I actually said it aloud to Tim: "I'm sorry, but I do NOT want you to remarry. I do NOT want you to be with any other woman for the rest of your life! I just want you to think about ME after I'm dead." Well, what does a husband say to that? I think Tim said something to the effect that I was not going to die and we didn't need to worry about that at the moment. Thank heavens we got off that train of thought.

After about a week in the hospital, a psychiatric nurse appeared in my door. Here was a person who was a breath of fresh air. She was smart, funny and had a matter-of-fact attitude along with some genuine sympathy for my illness. Such an approach enabled me to accept her suggestions. Apparently the nurses had observed my plummeting spirits, and after talking with my doctor, decided I might need a different kind of help.

Looking back, it seems absolutely essential to me that a psychologist or counselor should be a mandatory part of the initial evaluation. A patient is seen by a nutritionist, a pharmacist, a financial person, a social worker and a team of doctors, but not necessarily by a mental health person. And yet, if ever one's mental health is in jeopardy, it's when they are told they have cancer! After a few discussions with this psych nurse, we decided I should try some medication for anxiety. I was resistant at first. I had never been one to choose drugs or to let a doctor medicate me if I thought there was a more "natural" way, like diet or exercise. But the nurse explained, in detail, how "serotonin blockers" work and why I was an ideal candidate. This differed greatly from being told that I was depressed and needed Prozac, as I had been told twice before. In this specific situation, I had very real reasons for anxiety. So, we commenced with a small dose of an anti-anxiety medication, and within five or six days, I began to feel a difference. It wasn't a radical change, just a shift in my focus, as if a veil of darkness had been lifted. Rather than seeing everything through a dark lens of despair, I could see things more rationally.

The chemo had done its job after days of continuous IV and finally the nausea and aches and pains took hold. Pain medication was needed often and my appetite was reduced to zero. Food was a constant challenge; just to think about it was difficult. As a person who loves to eat, this new state was like being in a foreign, and hostile, country. Liquid nutrition in a can became my lifeline. I lost 12 pounds in the first 16 days of my stay and soon my hair began to fall out.

In anticipation of the "fallout" I had my hair cut to about an inch in length the first week in the hospital. My scalp had become very tender to the touch and after a few days of a tingling sensation, I was sitting in bed and I saw a clump of hair on the bed. I reached for a hank of hair and it came out in my hand. I had, at the time, two dear friends from Chicago visiting and they were taken aback by my cavalier attitude about my hair. "Let's wash my head in the sink!" I said excitedly. "Let's get all this hair off!" My friends looked confused, even worried, "Janno, are you okay?" one of them asked. "Yes! I've been waiting for this. Let's get it going!" And so we did. We scrubbed my head with shampoo in the sink and clumps of hair came falling out. The problem was that not all of it came out, so when we were finished, I still had sprouts and tufts of blondish fuzz in random spots all over my head, sort of like a baby duck. It was not my prettiest look, but what the hell? I just felt that it was another hump I had gotten over and we were on our way to recovery. Every step that happened brought me closer to completion of the whole process; that's what I thought at the time. Even the grueling nausea, the difficulties of wrecked "plumbing", the papery texture of my skin; all of this seemed to be right because it was exactly the way it had been described to me. I knew it was coming and since it was there, I felt I could get through it and be closer to my goal: healing.

I tried to walk a little bit in the halls everyday. I would push around my IV pole after donning my protective garb: a cover for my head, covers for my slippers, a hospital gown over my pajamas, surgical-type gloves and a thick mask called a duckbill mask. There is a reason it is called a "duckbill"—it looks like one. So out into the hall I would traipse, trying to think about Lance Armstrong and his courageous battle. He had been treated in this very hospital; his spirit was there. I imagined that he probably didn't lie in bed all day. But it was hard to get myself out the door, it was hard to shuffle along, and it was just so strange and sort of demoralizing to find that even just walking was difficult. Once, when Lucas was visiting, I went out for a walk, determined to show him how well I was doing. I got about halfway around the bend in the hallway and I started to feel light-headed and weak. Lucas had gone to refresh my water jug and so I called for a nurse. She made me sit down and called for a wheelchair to take me back to my room. I started to weep, out of embarrassment and despair. I didn't want Lucas to see me that way. I was trying to choke out that explanation to a nurse when Lucas came back in the room with my water. He asked what was wrong and I told him I didn't want him to see me so weak; I was his *mother*, I was supposed to be there for *him*. He sat down on the bed with me and put his arms around me. He said he didn't think I was weak; in fact, he thought the contrary. Whoa, that was really something—to be comforted like that by my son, my very grown-up and compassionate son, in a reversal of our roles. What a guy.

I don't know, to this day, whether or not there is a special philosophy at IU Med Center that promotes positive thinking on the part of the caregivers. From the moment I arrived on 5-N that fated night of Feb. 16, every single person I talked to said, "You can beat this. You are young and healthy and you can get through this." There was one resident in particular, a young woman I only knew by her first name of Chadya, who saw me crying as I waited for the attendant to wheel me down to an x-ray, and she kneeled down next to me and said, with her gaze riveted to mine: "You will beat this. You are young, and healthy and strong. I can see how strong you are. You will do this." So I never doubted it. I didn't know much about leukemia when I started the whole thing, but as I learned more, I believed I would be on the winning side of every percentage that I read about. I would be the one statistic that would be a survivor, a victor in this battle. Every nurse, every technician, and every doctor (and there were many, given it is a teaching hospital) gave me the same upbeat attitude, and so I matched mine to theirs, and together we would heal me.

3

T*he primary doctor who oversaw my care* was Dr. Larry Cripe, a hematologist. I remember hearing his name when I was first admitted and wondered when I would see him. I had begun my treatment with the resident team and heard his name often in their conversations. I knew he was the head of the Hematology and everyone spoke of him with respect and reverence. When he finally arrived in my room, I said, "Ah-hah, the mysterious Dr. Cripe." And he replied, chuckling, that he didn't think he was all that mysterious. He came over to my bed, eschewing the mask and gloves, shook my hand and focused his eyes on mine. Right away, I felt that he was interested in me the person, rather than just me the leukemia patient. He asked all about my family, my lifestyle and my work. He was intrigued by the fact that Tim and I were actors and artists, and especially interested to find out that we lived on 80 acres out in the country. He saw my photos of our farm and my family and friends and horses and goats and cats that I had posted up all over my hospital room. He looked at one picture of me feeding our goats, and asked, "Is that where you live?" I said yes. He said, "Well, we need to get you back there." That was his mission: to get me back to my life.

Aaah, my life. What was my life? I was trying to remember how I was in that "other life". I had always been a busy person, a "do-er". I always have thought that it is important to be involved, so I was often running from activity to activity, driving to soccer practice, and volunteering at the schools, and working as an actress whenever I could. I taught writing workshops here in town, and occasionally traveled for an acting job out of town. I was a wife and a partner to Tim. I had learned to sing with him and performed in concert with him whenever I could. I often describe myself as a "co-dependant singer" because I really can only sing with Tim. Singing with Tim is such a natural part of our life together; we sing at home, we sing in the car, we talk about singers and songs we like, our kids talk about music they like. We're also great collaborators in writing songs. I have no ambitions to be a singer on my own; my own creative life is full enough. But I love to be a part of it and it works for us.

Our marriage had been through some rough spots but we had come out on the other end stronger than before. I loved being a wife, I loved being a mother, I loved my life with all its chaos and craziness. Where was that person, that me? I began to review that "old life", as though looking at snapshots in an album, so I could place myself in some context other than that of a cancer patient in a hospital. My "old" life felt like a different country I had lived in long ago, and I wondered if I would ever return. But with the cards and letters and especially e-mails coming in, I was reminded of my life out there, a number of lives actually; distinct periods of time when I lived in a particular place or worked at a certain job, or had one child, then another, then another. There were many chapters to review. Much of it came rushing in through the website.

The love that flowed through all the messages was palpable. I felt a surge of energy when I read them or listened to them, especially when I was feeling crummy. I remember one particularly dry-witted friend who wrote about a friend who, just as he was about to be broadsided by an SUV, thought to himself, "Oh boy, this is going to be inconvenient." He thought I must feel the same way! "Inconvenient" indeed. One day I tried to write an update on the journal page. I had Lucas set the laptop up for me and this is what I wrote:

> Hi everyone I am a little fuzzy from the Atavin but I'll see how this goes. The morning brought news of another hip biopsy so that was fun but I gripped the doctors hand so hard that she said the chemo hadn't affected my strength. So now we're waiting to hear if I need more chemo or not, I am starting to fall asleep...bye love Jan and tell everyone how much I love the e-mails and the cards and every bit of love I have I send right back out for that's the way it works

I have only a vague memory of actually writing those words but I do remember that I felt as if I had been given permission to say what I really felt, without censoring myself. Obviously punctuation didn't matter, but more importantly being "reserved" or "polite" didn't matter either. I just said what I felt.

So the chemo did its job and wiped out all my fast-growing cells, which include not only leukemia cells but also those of mucus membranes, hair and skin. Now I had to wait for my white count to come back up and this stage of the treatment often involves some transfusions of red blood or platelets. I had received a number of blood transfusions, but on March 1, I had an interesting experience with the platelets. I have to say, every single time I would get blood and the nurse would hook up a bag of the bright red liquid, I felt immense wonder and gratitude for the donors out in the world who were giving me such a gift. They had no idea where their blood would go and anonymous patients, like me, were the lucky recipients of their generosity.

On one particular day, I was to receive platelets. These come in an IV bag, a pale yellow substance, hooked up like any IV, about which I was now an old hand. I decided to take my pole and go for a walk, all the while the platelets were drip-dripping into my veins. I was feeling rather proud of myself for getting out and walking. My friend Jennifer had come from Chicago to spend the night with me, and we were chatting as we walked and I felt pretty good. We returned back to my room and just as I sat on the bed to take off mask and booties and gloves, I felt an odd sensation. It started slow, like a few ants crawling on my arms. Then it increased, to my neck and my stomach. I started to scratch. Within one minute, my whole body was itching, as if I was being eaten by little bugs or tormented by nettles. I began to scratch at myself furiously and panic at the same time, because it was such an overwhelming sensation. Jennifer buzzed for the nurses and when they saw what was happening to me, they administered a high dose of Benadryl, right into my lumen so it went into my blood stream instantly. I have never been able to take Benadryl pills because they make my head feel weird, like the top is coming off. But I had not considered it an allergy, so I hadn't mentioned it. Suddenly, the room began to spin and I felt as if I was going backwards in a long tunnel. I couldn't hear what people were saying and I held onto Jennifer or my nurse Kim as hard as I could, fearing if I let go, I might die. I could feel the darkness of the tunnel closing in around me and I felt like I was passing out. I remember having the distinct thought that I had to go out the other way, toward the light. So I willed myself to breathe and to get out of that bad place and I began to slowly calm down.

I didn't know at the time that Jennifer was extremely wary of hospitals and the whole episode was testing her mettle. At one point (she told me later) she had to let go of me and go sit down to catch her breath and let the blood go back to her head, only to step back into my delirious steel grip moments later. It turned out to be a journey for both of us, rewarding in that crazy kind of way.

The doctors administered Tylenol and Atavin as a way of calming the inflammation, and after three hours of slow breathing and packing my legs with ice, the itching subsided. That was when we realized that I would always need pre-medication for any blood products, like hemoglobin, platelets or transfusions.

A word about the nurses: I have seen my share of nurses in my adult life. Of course, with the births of the three boys, but also with Connor's surgery and also with my parents' various medical situations as they grew older and sick before they died. I have always been aware of nurses and the jobs they do in a peripheral sort of way. But I never stopped to consider what oncology nurses must face; what they have to know, what they deal with, how much people depend on them. Most of the nurses at IU Med Center were women, as is still common these days, but I was attended to by three or four male nurses during all my days there. They were great guys, all very knowledgeable and as capable as their women counterparts, and some of them would pat my shoulder in a gesture of kindness when they were in my room. But there were a couple of times, when I was feeling so much despair, loneliness, anger or grief just to name a few of the more outstanding emotions, that it was the women who embraced me. Physically, with their arms and their hands, and chests and strong bodies…they sometimes used all of them to hold me. I once called the nurses desk at about 3:00 in the morning and the nurse on call came in. She was a darling young girl, with pierced tongue and groovy make-up and hip clothes, a little alternative, just ever so slightly "goth" and she was extremely competent with all the changing of my IV tubes and administering medications. But at this hour of the morning, I needed to be held. Here I was, a 52-year-old woman, and she was in her twenties. She was bustling around, doing her job, and I worked up the courage to ask her if she would sit on the bed next to me. I was a little embarrassed but I asked, "Can you hold me? I mean, really, like, give me a big hug and not let go for a little while?" She didn't miss a beat. She just said, "Sure" and plopped down next to me on the bed and held me, rocking slightly, for a long time. In that moment, she was a mother to me.

On another occasion, early in my first stay, I had overwhelming sadness in the middle of the night and buzzed the nurses' button on my bed. A very young woman entered, turned out she was a student nurse, and I skipped any preamble and just went right to weeping. Barely able to take a breath, I asked her to please, please explain why leukemia happens, why cancer happens, why it happened to me. Poor thing, she was absolutely taken aback and very gently and apologetically asked if she could go get her supervisor. I felt a little silly as she returned, superior in tow, both of them looking stricken as to what they might find. The supervisor had thick gray hair and an air of wisdom about her. She exuded warmth and compassion, and sat on the side of my bed for an hour, listening, nodding, touching my hands, my face. I gradually calmed down and could actually talk and give voice to my fears. She held me and said she understood. She said it was good to talk about it and good to cry and that was all healthy and part of the process. She said I had to grieve, that it was only natural. The younger nurse just watched. A few days later, the supervising nurse stopped in my room and told me that what had happened that night was one of the best things that could ever happen for a student nurse. She learned volumes that night, about being a patient, about being a nurse. She smiled at me and said we had all benefited.

There are elements of being a patient in the hospital that make you feel like a child. Just being at the mercy of the doctors and nurses and other caregivers makes you feel little. And that can be a very good thing. It means you can ask questions like a child, unafraid and uncensored. It means you can ask for hugs or massages or foot rubs or to have your hair brushed or played with (if you have any hair) or have lotion rubbed on your back or arms—the kind of stuff your mom did for you when you were little. It's time for that again, when you're in the hospital. Of course, it's time to be strong and brave too, and to ask questions and be involved in your medical situation. BUT, allowing time to be nurtured and cared for was one of the most helpful discoveries for me—getting hands-on care, not just medicine. The hardest part is asking for it.

A community began to develop on the website. People started to write each other, and refer to each other's e-mails on the site itself. It became (and still is, as of this writing) a network of friends, of people reaching out to each other and everybody seemed to be getting something positive from it. Some people were writing in from places as remote as Iceland and Uruguay. Others, not to be outdone, wrote from fictitious places, like the Great Wall of China, or a boat on the Nile River, as if they were there.

It was true; my friends were wordy, thank God. Writers started to come out of the woodwork. Many of the people that I had never known to be eloquent became so, and profound and poetic. It was as if this illness was giving us permission to say things we had always wanted to say but hadn't, or couldn't, for whatever reason. Our friend Mary, from Detroit, became known for her fabulous taste in poetry and her, sometimes daily, contributions of a new poem were cause for joy. The world was getting smaller as everyone gathered to help me heal, and to help each other face the specter of illness and possible death that was not far behind in everyone's minds. People also wrote about the daily details of their lives, and I loved that. I loved hearing about the comings and goings of the people I knew. I got descriptions of grocery shopping trips, complete with the list; I heard about the new restaurant coming to town (will it last? It's not a chain…who knows?) I was quoted lyrics from songs, poems, children at the elementary school were writing poetry, as I had taught them a year before, and those verses were coming over the e-mail. It was a veritable fount of information.

Many people, knowing that I am a Unitarian, were very careful to include all the deities they could remember, or encompass all the traditions of prayer and meditation. Others just embraced me into their own religious beliefs, knowing it was the very best thing they could do. I felt nourished by all expressions of faith, and was deeply moved to be held in the prayers of the B'hai group here in Columbus as well as a Lutheran church in Kentucky as well as the Episcopal Cathedral in New York City. I was being prayed for and meditated on by people of many faiths and I honestly felt carried along by the energy and the love. This was really happening and I was lifted up.

Friends were writing on the daily journal, because most of the time I was not able to.

SUNDAY, FEB. 27—To all Jan's friends and family, first of all, she looks fabulous. My joke for the day was that Jan looked better after a week on chemo than I did after a night on her sleeper Blue Chair! And it is true. She is having dreams about her room and she keeps thinking the room has changed or that she has moved to another one. The things that keep her located where she is are the photos of all her friends and family so if you have any pix of yourselves with or without Jan, send them along. Her room feels like a healing place. She finds herself being drawn to soft colors: pink, lilac, yellow. She tried a black pajama top on and thought she looked like the "Grim Reaper" (her words—ha ha). She is pretty thin and pale so the brighter colors seem to boost her spirits. Everyone that I have met, all the doctors and nurses, therapists and support staff are wonderfully kind and spend as much time with Jan as she needs, answering questions and giving support. Keep those prayers coming. I'm sure they are working. Love, Janet

WEDNESDAY MARCH 2—By now you've read the best news of the past 14 days (has it only been two weeks? This seems like a lifetime) Jan's bone marrow biopsy came back clear today! No signs of leukemia cells, so she will not have another round of chemo right now. She will be pumped with good blood-building substances to help healthy cells grow and return her immune system to "normal". Jan is celebrating tonight in fluffy new jammies, wrapped up in a fluffy soft blanket all delivered by our favorite shopper, Sue T. Jan's companion this evening is her ever-faithful friend Liz. Tonight's menu featured a burger, cooked in the sterile kitchen for neutropenic patients, followed by a lovely selection of germ-fighting pills and nausea reducing substances. No morphine drip tonight—hooray! Jan said her "chemo-brain" is making it impossible for her to read. Is she just making excuses for becoming a "West Wing" fanatic? Perhaps, but nevertheless, refrain from sending books until she can enjoy them while sipping tea on the veranda, Jack and Connor playing on the swing overlooking the hill in the backyard, after having Tim play a tune for her…that will be the time for books! -Julie

It was a time for rejoicing: clean bone marrow. My friend and resident under Dr. Cripe, Dr. Johnny (a young woman), requested that she be the one to come in and tell me. She said, "I've had to bring you so much unpleasantness, I really wanted to bring you some good news!" It was great news. It was an indicator that my body, that the leukemia cells, responded. They could be killed. It seemed, in my mind, like a battle had been won. But I knew it was far from over.

So a new phase was beginning. Now that my blood needed to replenish and the cells needed to get to work, all I could do was wait. My daily team of doctors was now headed by Dr. Mehta who explained that I needed to get my "neutrophils" to a certain number. Neutrophils are the big white blood cells that fight infection. When you don't have them, you are considered "neutropenic" which indicates your immune system is very compromised. Stimulating their growth would be accomplished by taking daily injections of "Nupogen" a stimulant of such cells, and transfusions if needed, and waiting. The thought of waiting and waiting drove me a little crazy. I wanted a task, a way to grow these things.

I have never been good at waiting. I roll up my sleeves and say okay what should we do here? I wished it was like a garden because then I could go out with my shovels and hoes and prepare the soil and rake it and make my furrows and mounds and plant seeds—I do know how to grow things. But growing blood is different. All I could do was to let the bones do their secret work, get enough rest, and try to get enough nutrition in me, which was particularly hard because everything tasted like metal. I told Dr. Mehta that I was going to talk to my bones and he didn't laugh. He said, "If I were you, I'd talk to them everyday." He told me that the bones that were doing the work were my hip bones (there's some substance, as Tim used to joke), pelvis, collarbone, sternum and skull...these are the sites of adult blood production. I figured those childbearing hips of mine would have sufficient bone mass to produce enough blood for all of me.

I wished I could say that I was charging into this battle with my face to the sun. The fact was that I was extremely mercurial and emotional and sometimes it just hit me like a ton of bricks that I was there in that hospital room with this "thing". Even with a team of doctors and nurses and a veritable community of support rallying around me, I knew at the end of the day that I was alone with my leukemia. I wanted to be brave. I wanted to be heroic. But there were times when I was stymied. That's when I would cry a lot and mess up my sinus infection and become completely congested and feel even worse. It was a vicious cycle.

As one might predict, the staggering cost of my treatment was beginning to be evident in the bills that arrived in the mail at home. I didn't see them, thanks to Tim, who filed them in a large plastic bin. But the insurance policy that I had at the time was through the Screen Actors Guild, one of the actor's unions of which I was a member, and they were stepping right up with notices of my eligibility and payments that would be made. The irony of this is that I was eligible for that coverage because of a commercial I had made the year before. It was a high budget commercial that I had shot in Napa Valley for a whole week and the residuals had been most welcome, especially to a couple of actors used to more humble salaries of the theatre. The product that I was promoting? A post-chemotherapy <u>cancer drug</u>, one that I actually never used, but that commercial paid for the first year of my treatment. Insurance problems would raise their ugly heads later down the road, but for the time being I was grateful to the powers that be for casting me in that commercial. Who knew...?

4

A significant thing happened to shape my hospital experience. Three or four different people had sent me paper and colored pencils. I had put them away in a drawer at first. Then one day, I decided to take up one of the pads of paper and scribble a little. I had no idea what I would draw, or if I would want to even try. But there was something about the medium, the feeling of pencil on paper, the immediacy of something appearing; something about all of that appealed to me. It used a part of my brain that was not too taxing; yet it stimulated me. I had done some drawing in high school, but it had been a long time since I had any thoughts of creating visual images. My medium of choice for the last twenty years had been acting in the theatre, and then writing. But I could not focus enough to write. The occasional entries in the web journal were all I could muster. So the stars were in alignment, I suppose, as I picked up the pencils and began to draw, for that became a life-changing activity for me, a way to express myself that was simple and straightforward. My drawings were certainly simple, especially at first. I drew myself as a stick figure in various hospital scenarios. I appeared as a bony, bald and often blue figure. I don't know why I portrayed myself as blue, but from my perspective today, I think it was subconsciously metaphoric: I <u>was</u> blue. Not only was my skin a grayish-blue, but I had a case of the blues.

I became bolder and more confident as I went, beginning to use more color, more detailed imagery, and I started to feel freer about it, so much so that I started to show my drawings to people.

The nurses were the first to see what I was doing. Nurses are on the frontline; they <u>know</u> what's going on by being with the patients all day or all night. They are the ones coming and going from the room for hours on end. They are observant and vigilant and they are aware of the little nuances in behavior or conversation. So they caught on right away to the fact that I was suddenly occupied with something and asked to see what it was. I was reluctant at first, but then I showed them some of the pictures. The nurses were so excited to see that I had found an outlet for myself, a way to cope with all that was going on. They encouraged me to continue, and to put the drawings up on the walls. Soon the doctors were inquiring what I had I drawn lately, and how was the artwork coming. My primary doctor, Dr. Cripe, took an interest in my artwork. He would discuss the pictures with me, and make comments and give critiques (often pointing out my difficulties with perspective—I would defend myself, "I <u>know</u> that head is too big for that body but she's laying down!"). We had talked about plays and poetry and now we talked about my drawings. How cool and unbelievably lucky for me to have such a doctor! The whole picture of healing was big enough to include my artwork and literature and conversation, and for that I was grateful. Our friend, April, came to take pictures of the artwork and she posted them on the website. That was the beginning of my "Leukemia Art".

By about week 3, there were many conversations going on among the friends of the website. There were various discussions about Maija's cookies, which were becoming legend as the tales of their wonder circulated amongst everyone. Then Sara wrote with many contributions from and about her seven-year-old Sam. Our friend Janie, a casting director in Chicago, kept us all abreast of film and TV goings-on in Chicago. We heard who was having lunch with whom, who was reading what and what movies were the best. People's kids and dogs and cats got into the news and there was a whole community of websiters that kept me afloat with their humor and insight. I could just picture them all out there in their lives, their ups and downs. I was a part of their lives just as they were a part of mine. It was so reassuring: I was alive, they were alive; the whole thing was a miracle.

Then I put a call out for jokes. I knew all about the "laughter is the best medicine" theory and I decided I could handle it, without hurting my chest or tummy too much as I laughed. I had no idea how far-reaching that request would go. The jokes started coming in from all points of the globe, from people I didn't know, and the word just kept flowing outward and outward, with nothing but the best wishes and concern and love coming back at me. They were also making each other laugh. I was, at times, a spectator to all the activity and I loved it.

I remember one morning I woke up panicky and thought, *I can't believe I have to spend another day in here.* You would think I'd have felt like that sooner (22 days thus far), but actually there had always been something interesting to think about or divert me from the monotony…or else I was in such a morphine haze, that I didn't notice where I was and that time was passing. The days just flowed by and I lost count. I was almost like an observer at times, watching myself go through the motions, like an actor in a surreal film; foreign probably, with a language I couldn't really understand.

So that particular day just carried on, with interesting moments and visitors and a big fat two-hour nap, and I got through it without going stir crazy. Then the docs were coming by and as usual they said, I was "doing great" and I said "If I'm doing so great, where the heck are the neutrophils?" Dr. Mehta said I was on Day 20 since the chemo started and they didn't expect to see neutrophils until Day 25-28 so he was not worried. (Good for him—of course, I figured I would be a new statistic and show neutrophils by Day 21, at least.) One night, a nurse told me I was the wellest sick woman she'd ever seen. *Bah humbug*, I thought. *Does that get me home???*

On a more sobering note, Dr. Cripe came by with his fabulous nurse, Sheryl (so smart and articulate AND she goes to the theatre regularly; in fact, she had actually seen me on stage at IRT before—small world) to explain the future plan. It seemed to be much more rigorous than I had anticipated. There would be at least two more biopsies and the possibility of another drug eventually if I were selected for that part of the clinical trial I had enrolled in. Yikes. Sheryl looked me in the eye and said, "You are fighting for your life here." Which certainly brought the gravity of the whole thing home. The vast onslaught of information was sometimes overwhelming, and in order not to go absolutely nuts, I had to just take one day at a time. Otherwise I might have exploded with all the what-ifs and maybes. I have never been so good at being in the moment. I am always ten steps ahead of myself, imagining the next new thing, and full of anticipation of how it's going to be, so staying with the reality of this thing was challenging to say the least.

Finally nausea was starting to be under control, and occasionally I could eat a bowl of cornflakes, but most of the time I could not choke anything down but the nutritional drink the hospital serves up. Chocolate only, thank-you very much. I was trying to grow the good stuff in my bones and in my blood and everyday I would whisper to my bones, "I love you."

I began to write more journal entries:

MARCH 11—Today is Jack's birthday. He's 11. My youngest son is 11? Yikes. I told him we would have to celebrate a little bit here, then when I get home, and then some more anytime he wants. It's also my sister Pat's birthday, and she's here! Some birthday celebrations we've been having. I had another allergic reaction to platelets today, in spite of the pre-medication. This time it started with my right eye itching and closing up and then my lips and nose swelling and stretching so that I looked like a putty figure gone awry. I told my sister and the nurses that my lips felt funny, but they kept saying, "No, it doesn't look so bad." But when I got up to look in the mirror, I could see that I looked like a troll. I was glad one of the doctors got up here to see it and when he walked in, he said, "Hi. Hmmm. You look different." Well, <u>yeah</u>. Anyway, the new pre-med cocktail is more cortisone, Tylenol and Demerol, which—can I say? Is just short of bliss. Less woozy than morphine and it just took the edge off…of EVERYTHING. I was so glad Pat was here and Cherry, one of my fabulous nurses, stayed longer than her shift, just to make sure I was okay. I'm telling you: the nurses here are miracles.

There were so many women around me. It just came naturally to them to nurture. The core group of women from my home town had a meeting at a local coffee shop every Monday morning to discuss what I needed, who was coming to visit me and when, and what did Tim and the boys need. Of course, casseroles and chicken dinners and box cakes started coming in for the boys. Rides were organized to help get the kids to soccer and basketball and band class. I figure, as I look back on their organizing and planning, that collectively they could run a Fortune 500 company without a problem. These women integrated my Chicago friends into the mix, dealt with my siblings coming in, and helped my boys with their homework. They cleaned the refrigerator and bathrooms and took in the mail. They covered every angle of this whole thing.

The men who visited were so dear. Lots of actors came from the theater and a few of my friends' husbands came, especially the more extroverted types. A lot of them didn't know what to say to me, and not all of them felt like they could touch me, so there was sometimes an awkward silence. Illness is a weird thing. It's hard to know what to say or do when you visit a sick person. I was learning not to take total responsibility for my visitors and not to worry if they were okay. It was finally sinking in that people really wanted to help me, and sometimes they needed to be told what exactly I needed. I almost always needed a foot rub. That was the easiest gift to take and the easiest for visitors to give and it connected us when we might not have words. Sometimes, a person just sitting in the room with me was the best medicine and no words were needed. James, my dear friend and playwriting mentor, my son Lucas, and of course Tim were the men who spent the night in the Blue Chair. The nurses were so impressed with them. They'd bring in sheets and pillows for the overnighters, and were especially solicitous to the men. "How sweet he is" my nurse Kim used to say about Tim all masked and gloved up to stay the night.

The artwork was building up a head of steam and so were my neutrophils. I was drawing everyday, and collecting a big pile of art that was exciting. And apparently, it was having a good effect on my marrow. The neutrophil count was on. One day, I had 4 neutrophils. Next day none. Next day 24. Next day none. Then I had 100. I was cautious to let this news out because, of course, it could go back to zero any day. So I was really happy, then serious again as I contemplated being disappointed. At a count of 500 neutrophils, the masks could come off and there was a chance they'd let me go home, with daily injections and blood counts twice a week. Tim and I had to meet with the doctors about home health care. I did have a triple lumen sticking out of my neck and it would certainly require some care—that would be another learning experience. I wrote:

MARCH 15—I'm hoping for a change in the weather. The thought of going out in this chilly gray weather freaks me out a bit. I am yearning for sun and sitting on the porch swing watching the boys shoot hoops and ride their scooters, although no sun on my bare skin. I've heard more and more about skin cancer these days—the last thing I need. I have to stay away from the barnyard and horse manure and hay, and I can't get elbow deep in the garden without my mask. I am dreaming of Spring and walking in grassy fields and sleeping in our bed and laying on our living room couch….ooh, now that's heaven! Every single person who has written or visited has helped me immeasurably…my gratitude is boundless, really. -Jan

WEDNESDAY MARCH 16—Okay, I was afraid to say it just in case it didn't happen but it did happen: neutrophils up to 300 yesterday and almost 500 today and they are letting me go HOME!!! Today!!! I am still a bit neutropenic, so I have to wear a mask in public. Then I come back in a week to see Dr. Cripe again in the clinic and probably have a biopsy. This will determine the next course of action: if I'm not in remission, I go for a bone marrow transplant. If I am in remission, I come back in a month for another short round of chemo, and then again another month later for another round. By then my skin, which has absolutely turned to parchment, may have recovered, and although I won't have hair by then, I will at least be used to being bald. I will keep you all posted on how it goes at home. This is leukemia…isn't it absolutely weird? But that's just the way it is. Love, Jan

The response was resounding: hooray, home sweet home! But I have to say that leaving the hospital was even more surreal than going in, if that's possible. I wept as I got dressed in my regular clothes that had been sitting in the closet all this time. I wept when they put me in a wheelchair and I had to say good-bye to the nurses, especially one of my most constant and wonderful, Mary H. I felt separation anxiety; who would help me, would we know how to do things, what if I can't do something the right way? The nurses are so competent and confident and they had been my caretakers for almost a month. I felt shaky and nervous to leave them. They all said that was perfectly normal; many patients have anxiety about leaving, but they pointed out that they were a phone call away, and I could reach someone at any time. They hugged me and wished me well, and I was wheeled down to meet Tim at the car.

Everything was so bright and stimulating, I had to shut my eyes halfway through the ride home. Then, of course, I got nauseated. We stopped at the pharmacy to get my boatload of prescriptions and whaddya know?! It costs a whole lot more to be sick out of the hospital than in it. The drug companies have us tied up in knots along with the insurance companies; who will pay for what, what new drugs are sky-high expensive until the developers lose the patent, etc. etc. It is a full-time job to figure it all out.

Then we drove up our lane and I was home. Home. Never has the word tasted so sweet. It looked so beautiful! And so different than I remembered it. Everything seemed bigger, like the kitchen cabinets and the doorways. The windows seemed so big and clean, and the view of trees and hills was breathtaking. No more air conditioning vents and rooftops of other buildings, which had been my view in the hospital. I felt almost drunk on the sounds and sights; what was once so familiar now seemed extraordinary.

That first night I felt so frail coming to bed. The face that looked back at me from the mirror was a strange one; a thin, gray, bald person. Was that me? But I had a great sleep in our own bed; no plastic crinkling sound from inside the pillow case, no clanking in the hallways, no nurse waking me up at 4 A.M. to take my "vitals". That night, I dreamed that I was asked to design a quilt…the women in the dream said, "We know you can't really sew but you have a great eye for design." So there I was, amongst these really great quilters who were looking askance at me, but I knew what to do. I was drawing some kind of big watery shapes in blue and purple and then I woke up and had to use the bathroom. And here's a bit of leukemia trivia: in the old part of the hospital where I had been ensconced, there were no bathrooms in the rooms, only "commodes", portable chair toilets. So can I say how great it was to come home and use a Flush Toilet??? It's sometimes the little blessings, you know? In the morning I awoke, surprised to find myself in a real bed, in our bedroom. I gingerly went down the stairs feeling like a stranger in my own house. Where I had once bounded down the stairs, I now stepped feebly, holding the railing, trembling slightly.

After the boys left for school, Tim bundled me up and we walked down our lane. There was so much sky and grass and wind—it was awesome. My legs felt like jelly, I was so Gumby-like. I sat down a few times, right there in the grass and felt the fresh air and thought I might weep for joy. I felt energized and alive, so very alive. I think that's a feeling that you realize after you've not felt alive; after you've felt depleted and on your way, possibly, to death. It seemed as if I had been on a road going one way and now I had taken a u-turn and began to go the other way. The way back, back to Life.

Then I came inside and thought I might unload the dishwasher, but just about collapsed. Back to the couch for me, where I would spend a great deal of the next month. I drew pictures and looked out the window and bundled up in blankets on the couch, happy to just watch everyone come and go, especially Connor and Jack. They were returning to an ease of being around me and they were so clearly happy just to have me home. I never tired of looking at my sons, and watching them, and sitting close to them so I could inhale their sweet smells. Every second was a gift, really. Every little thing seemed miraculous. Trees seemed so hugely majestic and astounding. The land spreading out beyond my windows seemed vast and almost incomprehensible, there was so much of it. My perspective was dramatically altered and happily so. I felt that nothing was worth arguing about, my desire for serenity and peace in our home was the ultimate goal—why not? Life is too short for bickering.

I remember one evening Tim and Jack and I were going to watch a DVD in our basement. We had finished dinner, Connor was doing homework upstairs, and we three sat on the couch to watch. I was sitting between Tim and Jack, and I began to feel a strange sensation. I felt as if the leukemia was trying to find me, or that there was a presence in my bones that was talking to me, distracting me from the movie. I began to sweat and fidget, until finally I had to jump up and move to the other couch. Both of the guys looked at me quizzically, wondering why I had moved. I mumbled a few words about being hot, and turned back to the screen. But I felt as if something was growing in me, that something was taking me down, away from my family, and I couldn't let them see. I felt like I was suffocating and that the knowledge of my disease was almost strangling me. I couldn't look over at my husband and my youngest son; I would weep. It was a strange and terrible thing to feel so "inhabited". We finished the movie and I slowly followed them upstairs, then to our room. I said to Tim that something had happened to me down in the basement. It was potent, like a sign. I knew that I did not want, or more accurately would not LET, leukemia take me away but the disease had a voice or a pull, like a magnet. It was a confusing experience. I couldn't tell if I was strong, or if leukemia was stronger.

I had never been a napper until then. My place on the couch was always warm, with occasional leave to walk outside. I had my drawing materials at hand, the phone, a wide variety of medications, a bottle of water and the ever present nutritional drink that kept me strong as I was learning how to eat again. I loved getting phone calls, but I am told I fell asleep on many occasions as people were talking to me. I was, for the first time in my whole life, feeling comfortable doing nothing, trying to just nurture my body with rest and care. I had permission to do this: the "leukemia card" we came to call it. "Mom's pulling that leukemia card again," the boys and Tim would say if I couldn't get up and do things. It was great to laugh about it and find humor in the disease. I started to talk about the disease in very irreverent ways, much to the surprise of some. Cancer, the "C word", is a big taboo in many circles of conversation. Even survivors don't often like to talk about it. Not me. I wanted to talk about it because I thought the whole thing was rather fascinating and I also felt relieved when I could speak about it. It felt as if I was de-electri-fying it, taking away some of it's power. I also felt that it was a way to show my sons that I was not beaten down by the disease. "Hah. I laugh in the face of leukemia!" I could shout, hands on hips, like a super-hero.

Lucas, away at college, was somewhat removed from the imme-diacy of my situation. Connor and Jack, however, saw me in my most depleted state. I was skinny, bald, kind of pasty and gray, and I had very little energy. Not the mom they remembered from a few months ago, not their usual mom. So I watched them for signs—I encour-aged them to sit close to me and just read or watch movies, or just hang out. They were conflicted, I think, about how much they wanted to take care of me, and how much they just wanted things to be the "old way".

One day, as I was hunched over my piece of toast that still tasted like cardboard and sipping my nutritional drink, Jack was making himself some scrambled eggs. I could hardly look at the food because I was nauseated still, but I was making an effort to sit at the table with him. I watched him cook, my eleven-year-old, seriously stirring the eggs, his yellow blonde hair framing his lightly freckled face. He looked up with his sad blue eyes, and asked me if we were ever going to have people over to our house again. I told him of course we would, but that I had to get stronger and healthier first. He said that Dad could do it all, make food, invite people; I wouldn't have to do any-thing. I explained that Tim had so much on his mind that I didn't think entertaining was going to happen real soon. He slid down to the ground in a slump and wailed, "So we're never having people over again??" I called him over to me and made him sit on my lap; facing out of course, I didn't want to get too much in his face. I held him from behind, whispered into his neck, "This is really hard, isn't it? Having a sick mom is just not fun." He started to cry and he said, "I hate cancer. I hate hospitals. I hate this whole thing." And I said I did too. I said he had every right to feel crummy and that it wasn't fair that he had to have a sick mother and I didn't blame him one bit for being mad. It was like a cloud had passed over the sun for a minute, a little rain shower and then the sun came out again. Jack was happy again, finished his lunch with me and went out to shoot hoops.

Connor, on the other hand, was stoic, unemotional, and did not express much. But he would come and stretch out on the other couch across from me in the living room and read. At thirteen, he was already 5'11" with the longest legs in the family, and his dusty blonde hair straight and shaggy like an English rock star. He is more introverted than his brother, "reserved" we like to say, much like his dad. When I had been in the hospital, he was the one who was more comfortable there than Jack. The hospital made Jack jumpy and anxious. He'd want to go out and walk around, or go watch TV in the lobby. Connor would don his mask and climb into bed next to me, content to watch whatever I had on television or to read or just lay there listening to Tim and me talk. Maybe because he had been hospitalized before and knew what it's like to be sick, he had a very calm and relaxed attitude about my extremely passive state. He didn't expect much of me, at least outwardly, and I tried to make sure that I didn't just assume everything was fine. I tried to subtly check in with him now and again, and he'd always say he was "okay". I know it was hard for him too, though. How weird to have a mom on the couch everyday after school, one who didn't do any driving or volunteer with basketball snacks or come to soccer games. If I did go out, I had to wear a mask, and that was more embarrassing than not having me there at all.

There were some somber moments for Tim and me, in the privacy of our bedroom, after we shut the lights out downstairs and we were alone. Sometimes I would feel the sheer weight of the thing, slowing me down as I climbed the stairs to our third floor room. I'd sit heavily on the edge of the bed, just sit there as if frozen, hardly thinking, the inner voices in my head slowed to a trickle and I would just BE, sensing the world around me but not able to give it words. Tim would ask me what I was doing. "I don't know. Sitting." I'd say. He gave me room to articulate, if I could, and I often ended in tears, thinking about the fact that I could die. How would a future for our family look without me? It was as if I was missing them, and all the things that might ever be, already. If I was lucky, I would come around to a kind of peace, knowing we all are going to die, we don't usually get to choose our death, and the paths we are on are our own. My children's paths are their own; that was the hardest, knowing that I couldn't somehow control what their life would be like, their experience of me. I didn't want them to be kids whose mother died while they were still so young. But I had no power over that, and sometimes I could find peace. Other times, however, I fell asleep in utter despair.

Then there were the times that I'd be brushing my teeth and standing in the bathroom next to Tim, in my rather ravaged state, scrawny and bald and sort of grey around the eyes, and there we'd be! I would think, and usually say, "This is kind of interesting, isn't it?" And he'd say, mouth full of foamy toothpaste, "Yessshh, it really ish." And we'd laugh, and it WAS interesting. Amazing, actually, the whole thing.

One day, I had been sitting on the front porch swing, and I was bundled up so the sun wouldn't touch me, and I was swaying slightly. I felt a tremendous urge to walk down the steps and go stand on the ground. I wanted to feel my feet on the solid earth, to stand with the trees, the birds, the air, the sun. I looked around our land, out across the front field to the trees that were still bare, and around to the nearby branches where little birds were chirping, and I had to get up. Get up and go down the steps to the ground, to feel the earth beneath my feet, the air on my face. I wanted to lay down in it, to crawl in amongst the dried grasses and the pinecones on the ground, and feel the dirt. I have always had a "thing" for dirt—I love it. I am not afraid of it. As a child, I loved to play in it, to my mother's consternation, as I had permanent dirt on my knees and in my fingernails. I knew I couldn't really dig around in it in my post-chemo state, so I stood there in the beautiful air, with the sounds of birds and breezes filling my head, and I closed my eyes. Suddenly I felt a surge—a SURGE— of energy flow up through me! Like a rush from a shot of whiskey or something, it was there, flowing in me, up from my feet to my head. I remember it as if it was yesterday. Then I heard a sound I have learned to know since I have lived in the country: the cry of a red-tailed hawk. I opened my eyes and there he was, soaring above our field, probably hunting. I felt the earth tremble beneath me and flow through me and it was as if the universe was smiling at me and inside of me. I went inside with the confidence that I would be well.

5

I *wrote journal entries* as developments happened:

FRIDAY MARCH 25—Whew! So much to say!! First of all, I have to send out a huge and heartfelt thank-you for all who have donated to our Medical Fund. We are facing some huge bills and I can't say enough about how grateful we are. I am grateful for every line that has been written, every prayer, every visualization, every thought, wish, joke, poem or card that has come my way. I feel sure that it has all contributed to the next thing I have to say, which is My Big News: Yesterday I had my check-up with Dr. Cripe at the Cancer Pavilion and had a bone marrow biopsy. Thank heavens that Laura was with me to hold my hand because this one was deep and more painful than the last ones and apparently quite "thorough". It showed clean marrow and I am officially in remission! They want me back in the hospital next Wed. March 30 for another round of chemo. For what they call "consolidation" chemo, to get every last cell that might be hiding in the recesses of my bones. I will come home after that for three or four weeks and then go back to the hospital for yet another six days of chemo…and then, probably, I am done. Then it is watchful blood tests and 3 or 4 times a year of biopsy, then five years in remission are what is required to say one is "cured".

I am nervous but resolved about going back in. Now that I've been out and at home, I have such a different perspective on my time there. BUT, the fabulous nurses will all be there and I know I can count on every single one of them to take great care of me; they are all so nurturing and SMART!! I will have a different daily team of docs but Dr. Cripe will still be the main guy and I love him. I believe he and his team are, along with all of you, saving my life.

So, that's the scoop. It seems to be moving so fast now. I am really positive that this journey will end up in health and full life…I see no other way. Thank-you again for absolutely everything, -Jan

The days right before my return to the hospital were strange and full, in the anticipation of what was to come. I was scared but resolved to keep on the path that the doctors had spelled out so confidently. I had that fear sitting deep inside me all of the time, but rarely did I let it all out. If I did, it was privately, with Tim. I did not want the boys to be any more worried than they already were. We talked rationally about what was coming, and we all knew we just had to get through it. My friend Betsy was coming from Los Angeles to take care of the boys while Tim had to finish the run of his play in Syracuse. Many people asked me if I wanted Tim to stay home. They said that I should just tell him not to finish the job. But I knew it was the best thing for all of us to have him finish that commitment; both because we needed the money and his weeks of employment for insurance, and because he needed the focus, the feeling of finishing the piece he had worked so hard on. It was unfortunate it had to take him to another city, but I felt it was necessary for him to go. He drove me to the hospital on April 1, helped me get settled, and headed off to Syracuse. He went with my blessing.

It was so different than the first time I entered the hospital. This time, I was actually glad to see the nurses that I knew and even though I was apprehensive about the chemo, I was prepared for how I would feel.

The first step was to go to Interventional Radiology to have a Hickman Port inserted. This was different from the triple lumen I had previously. I remembered how intensely uncomfortable I had been that first time, and how afraid I was of everything. This time I knew to speak up, as experience had taught me: "I'm cold, I'm scared, help!" The nurses laid warm blankets on me, slipped a pillow under my head and began to thoroughly explain the procedure. The nurse explained the "cocktail" they would be using for anesthesia. The radiologist came in and made some sarcastic remarks about how he would have to be the one to do the procedure since his colleagues were slacking off. But I boasted that he was the lucky one: to get to work on me. Where did I get this chutzpah, this bravado? I don't know, but I have found that every time I speak up, either to make a request or make a joke or let the people know how I feel, it works wonders. It is a way to say, in so many words, "This is Me, this is who you are treating, not just an anonymous patient lying on a gurney, looking like any other patient." Such an approach opens up communication and that is one of the keys to getting through something like this—communication and being involved; not letting the whole thing just "happen" to you. I do remember, as the anesthesia began to work it's wondrous way of sedation, I turned to the nurse and said, "Do people often tell you that they love you?" "No," she replied, chuckling, "actually, they don't." "Well, I love you," I said loopily. "I love everybody in this room." Later, as I had been wheeled out into the hallway and was coming to, I found a sticky note on my blanket that read: "Nice working with you! -the I.R."

One fabulous bit of news was that I did not have to be restricted to the neutropenic diet of food prepared in the sterile kitchen. Rita, caterer and event planner to the stars in Chicago and my dear friend, came to visit with food. Good food and lots of it. I could also order anything off the regular menu, and I ordered pasta with shrimp and broccoli and pesto the first night. This was exciting for about two days. Then the chemo effects hit and my appetite went away—gone, gone, gone. Rita was in the hallway giving away food, to the nurses or anyone else who could eat. Because Tim was away, my friend Betsy came from California to stay at the house and help out with the boys. Liz took over as the main hospital visitor and advocate for me. She had to learn the care and cleaning of my port for when I would go home, and was the primary contact for all things medical. I realize now that I was beyond lucky, I was (and am) truly blessed to have friends jump in to help. There are all sorts of resources that hospitals have to help people, and they are to be used! Definitely. The fact that

I also had friends working with me made the whole thing easier.

An odd thing happened during this time. I developed a rash over my legs, arms, torso, and back. These were itchy bumps that looked like many mosquito bites very close together. They did not appear on my face, hands, or feet, so if I was wearing long sleeves and jammie pants, as I usually was, you couldn't see it. But I could feel it. And it was a mystery to all. The doctors thought it was a reaction to one of the chemo meds but it didn't really present itself the usual way. So we all just stared at it, and rubbed anti-inflammatory creams on it, and I tried not to think about how hideous it looked. Two dermatologists came in to look at it, and asked if they could take pictures. I said yes, but covered my face. I thought that it would be bad news if one of my kids opened a biology book one day and saw me there in a photograph, staring back at them, as an example of some horrible skin condition. The rather unusual thing about it was that it never presented on my face, hands, or my feet; it covered my arms, legs, torso, back—but clothing could conceal it and one might never see that I had this hideous bumpy thing going on. So, the days went by, this hospital visit was short and…well, not exactly "sweet" but certainly sweeter than the last one.

Being at home this time was different because I was giving myself injections in the thigh every morning, going through my lists of medications three times a day, and trying to figure out what to do about my skin. I was in limbo, because I knew the skin problem could curtail my treatment, and I was on a track of aggressive therapy because I was participating in a clinical trial.

The best thing about this time was the company of my sister Adele for a week and then my brother Mark for the next week. I was very sick and nauseated when Adele visited me and that was hard for her to watch. As she likes to remind me; she "saved my life" after the birth of my first child (okay, I was a little hysterical) and she wanted to do it again. But I couldn't really figure out what I could do to be more comfortable and the pills for nausea just knocked me out. On top of that, she got a dose of living in the country! We can laugh about it now, but it was really stressful at the time: the water line from the street broke not once, but twice, from construction on the county road. So we were without water for a time (which is scary when you have a recovering leukemia patient on your hands and everything is supposed to be sterile) and when it did return, a blast of sludge came through the faucet and we had to boil water for a day until the line was normal again. Then, unbeknownst to Tim or me, we were low on propane and of course, the tank ran dry during my sister's stay. Tim was in Syracuse, it was five in the evening and we discovered that not only did we NOT have water, we had no gas for cooking or heating the water, should it ever come back on. It is times like these when I am glad I live in a small city. A call was made to the propane provider and the situation explained; in other words, we pulled the leukemia card! But it was no joke; I was recovering from leukemia and we did have to have clean and hot water. The delivery person, who lives many towns away from us, made a special trip that night. My sister, who had never seen a propane tank filled, stood outside the back door calling encouragement to the guy while I stood inside the glass door and waved at him. I wanted him to see my scrawny bald self so he would know I really was sick. He was so happy to be able to help us. We, of course, were so grateful.

On top of all this chaos, the goats kept breaking out of the electric fence and our phone was not working properly. I overheard my sister describe the experience to someone on the phone: "Living out here is like camping or something!"

My brother Mark came in from NYC the following week, providing the boys with much needed male energy. He went to all their sports games and became a rabid cheering section at the handball tournament. One afternoon, he drove me out to the athletic field of the elementary school so we could watch the sixth graders, including Connor, sail hot air balloons they had made for a science project. We pulled up to the launching area just as Connor's balloon set sail. I stayed in the car because it was windy and cold, but Mark jumped out to cheer on his nephew in his loud and exuberant way. In minutes, a group of mothers had gathered around him as he regaled them with his charming ways and soon the teachers were looking his way. Everyone wanted to know who this cool guy was. "It's Connor's Uncle Mark!" In his five days with us, he made his mark at the elementary school and possibly, on all of Columbus.

Adele had told me a story about Mark doing his own gardening at his house in Connecticut. I don't know how she got this idea or why I believed her or even thought she would know about his gardening habits, but based on this information, I had a load of mulch brought over so Mark could spread it on the garden. He was clearly shocked at the idea that he would do any gardening. I told him, "Adele says you're really good in the garden." He looked horrified. "No way! I don't garden, I pay someone to do it." But he completed all of his outdoor tasks, griping and laughing all the way. Not only was there mulch to spread, which he did with Connor who was equally unenthusiastic, but there was a neighbor's borrowed tiller, with which I hoped he would prepare and turn the soil for a spring garden. This was definitely a time I wish I had taken pictures. Mark got behind the tiller, we turned it on, and there he went, lurching and bucking around the garden plot, grumbling and cursing. He was wearing nice pants and some kind of athletic shoes. I kept calling out, "Don't you want some boots?" "Nah," he grumbled, and went clomping along in the freshly turned soil, deeper and deeper into the dirt. I think it did him some good, underneath it all, to work the land.

One night, while Mark was doing the dishes after making us a steak and broccoli and salad dinner, which was amazing and delicious (amazing because I don't think I had ever seen him cook before and also because it was so tasty and the sheer fact of "tasting" amazed me). I was sitting in the living room while the boys were upstairs getting ready for bed. I happened to pick up some piece of literature about AML from who-knows-where and my eyes fell upon a particular statistic that was jarring. It related to people over fifty and recorded a low survival rate. I was stunned. I don't know if I had just MISSED this particular fact, but there it was, staring at me, and I felt like I was looking at my death sentence. I know many people are very interested in statistics, want to know the numbers, and the chances. I was not one of those people and it was really a mistake for me to look at this bit of info. But I had. I could hear Mark banging around in the kitchen—dishes clanking, the water running—and I couldn't move. I remember thinking that it was all futile, that all my forward thinking and action and positive outlook were for naught. Mark came out of the kitchen and said "Let's get you to bed." Off I went with those mind-numbing statistics in my head.

The next morning we dropped the boys off at church. I couldn't go in without a mask, and I was tired of looking like a sick person, so Mark and I went on a walk instead. We were walking in a small park nearby and I felt exhausted, like I couldn't complete even one turn around the small path. I held onto his arm and I could just feel a burdensome weight inside me and I knew it was because of what I had read the night before. I started out sort of joking, "You know…I read this weird thing last night." He was quiet. "Yeah, so I read that the statistics aren't so great for me, you know, my age, and stuff." I was trying to toss this revelation off like it was no big deal. He said, "To hell with the statistics, Jan. I mean, really. I have read so many horrible things about your disease that you shouldn't even be alive if you believed it all. That's the problem with the Internet: You read it and think it must be true. It's that old thing about if it's in print, we think it's true. But there are so many ways to have cancer, to have leukemia, and you're doing it your way. Which is NOT the way you read about last night. Look at you—you're doing great. You're a freaking miracle!" Now my brother and I are close, but it's usually through wacky humor or sarcasm or foul jokes, not being vulnerable and intimate. But this time I just fell apart and I cried in his arms right there on that sunny morning in the park. I held onto him and wept like I had never done before with him. He held on to me as tightly as I held him, and after a bit, I felt as if my troubles had passed for the moment and I was out of the woods. "Tears are God's antifreeze," I once read, and it seemed to be true.

By the time my sister Pat arrived, I was feeling better and could move around more. She was treated to a dose of teen angst as we drove first Jack, then Connor, to the school dance. We had to check back at the school to see how it was going, and then we had to make different arrangements for both boys. I think we made four trips back and forth to the school that night, Pat waiting patiently while I snuck in through the cafeteria to see how one boy was doing without letting the other one see me there. Over the next few days, we had a productive time cleaning out the refrigerator and the cabinets, replacing our ancient phone which had been driving all my caretakers crazy, and buying some loose linen pants for the warm weather ahead. I could not possibly think of shorts with the hideous bumps all over my legs, so long pants, long skirts, long underline_everything_underline for me.

All the love and closeness with my siblings was one of the great gifts of this illness. We all live far away from each other, in different parts of the States and it takes a lot to bring us together. Leukemia did that, and it's effect lasts to this day. We are closer now than ever.

The down side of my skin problem was the thought that the chemo hadn't really worked. One of the "Fellows" who worked with my doctor, in examining me first, said he understood I had "Leukemia Cutis" which means leukemia of the skin. I was startled to hear it had a name. But then Dr. Cripe came in with the whole teaching team, and when I said with some dismay that I didn't know I had "leukemia cutis", he glared at the student who had said that. Dr. Cripe assured me it was not a definite diagnosis and that we needed to wait until the skin biopsy and the latest hip biopsy results came in.

Waiting, again. It is REALLY hard to wait for a diagnosis. I had understood we would know by a certain time on a certain day and when that moment came and went, I was beside myself. Finally I had to call the nurse and inquire. "Oh no, it's not today," she said breezily. "We won't have the results for a couple of days." Aaaah! I had been agonizing all day, waiting for the moment when I would know if my treatment would radically change or we would proceed as planned. This was a day when drawing got me through. I sketched a very specific image of a woman waiting by the phone, hunched over and depressed. That was me.

Because of the skin condition, I was taken out of the clinical trial. It was such an odd sensation to walk around with this very uncomfortable, very sensitive skin rash. Although it was a sign that something was going on, nobody could pin it down with a definite diagnosis. It was decided that my brothers and sisters should be tested to see of they were a match for a bone marrow transplant…just in case. There are ten protein markers on the cells that need to be matched from the donor to the recipient. There are less than perfect matches in some transplant cases, but the aim is to find a perfect match. So we were starting the process even though we didn't know the results of the biopsies. Dr. Cripe had drawn me diagrams of the possible paths of treatment, and the line branched out into two paths at the point of "remission" and "relapse". Leukemia in the skin would mean relapse and we would skip the next round of chemo and go directly to Bone Marrow Transplant.

Bone Marrow Transplant. The very words gave me the shivers. I was only partially aware of the enormity of the procedure, but enough to be scared. When I would feel anxiety rise in my chest and throat as I pondered the possibility, I would try to quiet my mind. I wasn't always successful, but when I could breathe deeply, when I could relax and reassure myself, when I could just quiet all the fearful voices whispering like harpies in my head—then I believed in my recovery. I could really feel the strength of my body, the will to fight the disease, the powerful desire to live.

Someone asked me on the website how I wanted them to pray for me. I could only say, "However you want to…I'd like to be rid of this illness, but I am not sure it works that way!" I got a quick rejoinder from Heidi who said, "Ask for complete healing; nothing short of that." Okay.

Finally the word came that the bumps were not malignant and we were to proceed with the third course of chemo. I was so happy to hear the news that I was giddy. But I looked at the faces of the doctor and his nurse and they remained placid and calm. I had to ask, "Aren't you guys happy? I mean, I am really happy. Are you?" And Dr. Cripe said quietly, "Yes, we're happy." And I said, "Well, can I be wildly happy or do I have to be guardedly happy?" He said, "You go ahead and be wildly happy and I'll keep both oars in the water." I said, "You mean while I splash and flounder wildly about the pond, you'll stay in control?" "Yes, basically."

MAY 2—So we are dancing in the streets while Dr. Cripe stays the course. Thank heavens…someone has to be in control. They are working my chemo schedule out so I can be at my son Lucas' graduation from Earlham College next Saturday, a few days before I go back in. How cool!

And it was. It was a beautiful day and the ceremony was outside. My niece Jennifer was with Tim and me and we were standing up on our chairs, looking for Lucas as the grads came out. Suddenly I saw him, this handsome young man, smiling, confident, surrounded by friends who obviously loved him. I leaned out into the aisle just a little bit so he could see me as he walked by and grinned. Lucas motioned for me to take my hat off and I did. He gave me the thumbs up—I was as bald as a baby and he couldn't have been prouder. It was a fabulous send-off for the hospital. I went in five days later on May 12 and I wrote :

MONDAY, MAY 12—I have not been able to get online to write because our local dial-up service is so slow. I picture our dial-up as an office somewhere, in a basement probably, and it's dark and dank and some old guy is cranking a machine to get the computers hooked up—that's how slow our service is—but I digress…I am back in the hospital as of today. My first dose of chemo will begin in mere seconds. As I write Debbie (the fabulous Debbie of the very first night who explained leukemia to me) is hooking up a bag with the magic chemicals in it to my IV. She has to wear gloves while she does it because if she should get any on her skin, it would burn her. Oh great, what's it going to do to my stomach?? It was actually fun to see all the nurses today who have become my friends. I never thought I would actually be familiar with a hospital and comfortable in that environment. I guess you just never know…I will have six doses over five days and return home on the 17th. It's hard to come in knowing I am going to feel so bad in a few days, especially because I have been feeling pretty great. But I guess that's evidence of how quickly the body can repair and heal itself—what a miracle—and the fact that the rest of me is in good health. It has been such an amazing Spring and all the love love love that has been coming through these pages is healing me too. I am aware of the time this illness has taken and the stamina required to fight. It's actually interesting and unusual when it's new, but the whole thing is getting old. I'm sick of being bald and I am sick of the port in my neck and not being able to take a shower and the tenderness in my mouth…(whine whine whine) I am also aware of the stamina it takes to be a friend/participant in this whole thing…checking the website and staying interested in the recovery process and writing and just caring for so long because it is a long road and I have to thank you all for walking it with me. Okay, here it goes: drip drip drip into my veins. PLEASE let my body stay strong. Hey! I can have home made food again, and that is good news because, I swear, if the illness doesn't get you, the hospital food will…onward. -Jan

After one day of chemo, I could tell this time was different than the last. I felt absolutely slammed; every part of my body ached as though I had a bad case of the flu. The painkilling cocktail of choice was a combination of Tylenol, Atavin, and morphine—whew! Six days passed in a haze of pain and painkillers and riding the waves of nausea. This time I was aware of irksome things in a way I had not been before. My room was situated near the swinging doors to the unit, and every time someone would go in or out, the doors would go thump-bump-shump, in three parts. Thump-bump-shump; all through the night, thump-bump-shump…By the fourth day of my stay, I was having to control my desire to get the hell out of there. I think, in hindsight, that it was a good sign, a sign of readiness to go home. If I had to be in pain and nauseated, I'd rather do it at home. Of course, the schedule of the chemotherapy was the determining factor, and as soon as I had my last dose, I prepared to go home.

Indeed, home again on the couch was the place to be. All the green coming through the windows as May turned into June was positively nourishing, like a good meal for the eyes. The sight of buds on the trees and the little rows of beans coming up in my garden, courtesy of niece Jennifer when she had been visiting, were so encouraging. It was a cause for joy, these little visions of Hope; just the sight of things budding and growing made me think of the future. There <u>was</u> a future out there. All I had to do was get through this last phase of chemo and be on my way. Leukemia was just a blip on the big screen of my life.

I had to give myself shots of Nupogen again, to stimulate the growth of neutrophils. All my friends were now talking the lingo with me: lymphocytes, neutrophils, blood counts, etc. etc. Once again, we were cheering on the growth of the neutrophils and urging the blood to do the right thing.

Lucas had been holding down the fort while I was in the hospital and he remained the main chauffeur and chief bottle washer when I returned home…and my crossword puzzle assistant. Apparently this round of chemo really wiped out some cognitive brain cells. Basic language skills seem to have just evaporated. I stood in front of Connor one day with a small blue box in my hand and I asked him if he wanted this…this "thing"…this whatsitcalled…I absolutely could not find the word for it. My mind was a blank. (It was a Gameboy.) I was the source of much laughter with my inaccurate words and forgetfulness.

MAY 20—It has been determined that I should not answer the phone when I'm horizontal on the couch (command central of the living room). Apparently I had a couple of conversations yesterday that I don't remember at all and at one point opened up my eyes and saw a friend standing there. I asked her to rub my feet and that's the last thing I remember. I also was talking with someone on the phone and stopped mid-sentence until she yelled," Jan! Jan! Hang up the phone!" I guess it's exhaustion. I see this beautiful weather and I just want to be out in it and I think a little weeding or hoeing won't hurt and then I am flattened. It's not like being sleepy; it's like being emptied of all energy and strength. So…I will focus on getting full of energy and not empty and I guess that means more rest. Phoooey.
-Jan

That Spring, the weather was sweet. Just being home was divine. No matter how much I loved that hospital and the nurses, and no matter how well cared for I felt there, there was just nothing like home. The sweetness of my bedroom, the light coming in the windows, the comfort of the living room couch—all these conspired to heal me and replenish my strength. So when I went out to walk in the lovely air one day, I decided that I could walk out into the field a bit. My friend Mary who was visiting, called to me anxiously, "Not in the field, Jan, stay over on the lawn!" "Don't worry!" I said, "I'm not going far, just a few steps in to feel the tall grass…aaah!" I had stepped near a broken stalk of a dried weed, which pierced my skin ever so slightly, but as my immune system was compromised, my skin was thinner than usual and bled more easily. So I rushed inside immediately, washed it and put antibiotic cream and a bandage on it. No problem.

That was May 21. Then the morning of May 23, I went into town with Tim. I was wearing my mask and being diligent about keeping myself covered and clean. We were paying for our groceries at the health food store, when I told him I felt a little "off" and had to go home. By the time we arrived at home, I was feeling sort of sick, flu-like, and I lay down on the couch with a blanket. Tim had to go to the elementary school to drop off something for Connor, so I planned to rest until he came back. I began to have the strangest sensations. I was frigidly cold, wrapped up in two or three blankets. My teeth were chattering and I had this unbelievable thirst. I had a craving for soda, of all things. I bundled up and went out to sit in the sun and try to warm up. I called Liz and Mary and Cathy; nobody was home so I left them all messages asking if they had any sodas and could they come over with them right away?

I was finally able to reach Tim, who raced home. By the time he got there, Cathy had arrived with two Sprites, which I chugged, and Liz was on the phone to the Hematology clinic, telling them what was happening. We all finally realized this was something serious, and Tim picked me up (I couldn't walk) and scooped me into the car and drove me up to IU Med Center He found a wheel chair at the front door and took me up to 5-N. Dr. Cripe took one look at me and said, "Admit her." So I was back in the hospital, IV flowing immediately with antibiotics and fluids and vital signs being taken. All of my nurses and doctors were gathered around my bed as I began to vomit and sweat and moan. Dr. Cripe said it was a textbook case of infection, that it was being taken care of handily, but if we had waited another six hours, I could have been toast (my words, not his). What a scare.

MAY 24—So I'm back in the freakin' hospital! Much as I love this place, I'd really rather be home. I have a big infection and it is just disheartening to be here. The docs think it might be from that scratch on my leg from when I went walking in our field. Oh that makes me feel so stupid. Man, the lessons just get harder, not easier.

MAY 27—I am, again, waiting for neutrophils! I can't go home until I have enough of the little fellows, so send your prayers and energy this way once again. I can't believe that I am so used to being in a hospital and the sights and sounds and smells are no longer unfamiliar. It is a good place to be when you're sick, which I am, but I am sick of being sick and I am sick of being in a hospital so that makes for a cranky attitude…I am just ticked off. Yesterday I had another reaction to platelet infusion (3rd time) This time it was like mosquitoes all over my arms and legs, but no Benadryl this time so they just stopped the infusion until the reaction abated. I looked like a bear had mauled me, I scratched myself so badly. They put socks over my hands so I couldn't scratch, and I kept tearing them off. I was slightly crazed by the whole thing. I mean, you just lose your rational self in circumstances like that and the world goes topsy-turvy. It's a wild ride. Had to have more platelets though, so they medicated the hell out of me and I slept through the whole thing! So the platelets are in and doing their job and I am waiting for new blood to grow. -Jan

This was a terrible way to be in the hospital. This wasn't about leukemia, it was about treating an infection and I was mad at myself for being there at all. I was sick, really sick, for about five days and then my fever broke in the night I awoke the next morning feeling different.

This recovery was moving in such small increments (it seemed to me) but Dr. Cripe, in whom I had tremendous faith, said I was getting better everyday, he could see it. He has certainly seen more of this than me so I believed him. I was starting to feel better and I was so sick of this hospital food that I was WILLING the neutrophils to grow so I could get out of there.

The whole thing had gotten me thinking…(that's an understatement)…about how our bodies affect our minds and our emotions. This is certainly not a new thought. But I was experiencing it in a new way, new for me, that is. Once my body felt the littlest bit better, I felt more hopeful. Because I had been sick off and on for months, I was experiencing depression and despair. Illness is sometimes like a wet blanket, weighing a person down, making it difficult to get out from under. It was hard to be hopeful, hard to see the light at the end of the tunnel. And I began to think about all the people in our world with illnesses or chronic pain or long-term need for medications. Many of these are people in poverty, many don't have the resources to get the best care, and so how can they have hope? Yet our society expects them to function, to pull themselves up by their bootstraps, to get off their behinds and go to work? It is just so hard to be motivated when you don't feel good. I knew this was not new thinking but I was living it and so gaining a new perspective.

JUNE 1—This hospital stay has just entered the realm of the absurd. They are exchanging all the beds on the floor with new ones so there is wild activity out in the hallway. I begged the doctors to let me go walking out in the big hall instead of just on this unit (32 steps one way and 35 back) So I was out in the greater world beyond 5-N and I have to say, I probably look pretty bizarre in my gown, foot covers, gloves and "duckbill mask". There are beds crashing around and many groups of maintenance men moving them in and out of elevators and technicians showing the nurses how to use these high-tech beds and I am marching in and out of all of it, back and forth, back and forth. I finally got back to my room and there in the window, outside, was a window washer hanging from ropes, swishing his big brushes all over the windows. Then the guy arrived (late) with my breakfast just as a student nurse came in to practice doing an assessment: "Do you have any chest pain? Do you have any swelling? Do you have shortness of breath? How is your vision? Are you vomiting? How are your bowel movements?" Aaaaah, I NEED to get out of here. I suppose that's a healthy attitude to have. I have one more day, and then, with a promise to stay out of the garden and away from the barns, I can go home. One of the doctors said this could be a summer of going to museums, instead of being outside. She has no idea what's it's like where I live! Summer where I live is all about being outside, getting in the dirt, in the woods, in the water. It's all about swimming and gardening and having dirt under my fingernails from May to September. I guess this will be a different kind of summer. Okay, let's get these neutrophils up and running and let the summer begin! -Jan

The website was still humming with news from the outside—there was news of a friend planting heirloom tomatoes with names like "Vintage Wine, Amish Paste, Red Brandywine, Plum Lemon, Black Cherry, Paul Robeson"—how poetic! And news from the soccer field; it seemed that Jack was flying around as usual, even having a shut-out playing goalie, which he didn't often do and when he did, my heart was in my mouth the whole game. Apparently I had made an impression on the coach's wife (who was Jack's guardian angel as well as my friend) for she wrote that my rather loud and amazing whistle was much missed on the sidelines. (And I thought nobody noticed…)

Finally, I could leave the hospital and be at home. The nurses bid me adieu and said, "Don't come back!" I still required daily injections of antibiotics though, since I could not get them intravenously and they were not available in a pill. So I had to learn how to mix the antibiotic, a powder with sterile water, shake it, withdraw it into the syringe and push it into my port. It was daunting at first and my hands were shaking. Within two or three days, however, I was very confident and had to laugh at myself as I would hold the syringe up to the light and tap any bubbles out with my fingers. I felt like a real nurse! I would often joke with the boys as I did it: "I'm not a doctor but I play one on TV…" There was a sort of unreal quality to the routine because I never had dreamed I would become so knowledgeable about medical things and so fluent in the lingo. But there I was, talking about "flushing the line" and "changing caps" and "cleaning the site". Oh, we were all learning more than we ever imagined. Liz had become quite adept at changing the dressing around the port site. The hardest part was working with those damn gloves! It was summer and we were hot and she would have to get one glove on and keep the other one sterile, while putting the second one on, sweating and shaking and cursing like a bandit, and we would laugh at how many gloves we threw away. Tim became an expert too, as soon as we found gloves big enough for his hands.

6

I had been home only a few days when Tim announced he was taking me to Bloomington to get a "present". We had just celebrated our 14th anniversary on June 1 and he said he had a gift for me. I guessed and pondered and couldn't imagine why we would have to go to Bloomington to get a gift; what could be there? Then we went off the main road and took a turn up into the hills, towards the house of Dave and Krista, where Tim records and mixes most of his music. The whole thing became more mystifying; what could be at the studio that I could possibly want? I started to dread it; maybe this was a well intended, but misguided idea that Tim had. Oh, what could we be getting into? We drove up the hilly lane to the house and studio. Tim reached behind the car seat and handed me an animal collar. My first thought was: <u>a goat</u>. Dave must have a goat. We don't need any more goats! But that's weird, why would Dave have a goat? Well, it can't be a dog; Tim doesn't want a dog. But then Tim said, "There he is." And I looked out the window to see a shiny black Lab, wearing a rope collar around his neck and smiling and wagging his tail furiously. You know how dogs smile? Well, he smiled at me. Dave and Krista have about 4 or 5 dogs around all the time. I think there is only one dog that officially belongs to them, but it is dog heaven up there. This particular dog, however, was going to come home with ME. Omigosh! I had wanted a dog for years, ever since the stray that had found us a few years ago had disappeared. I had always had a dog in my life, but since we lost that little guy, we just couldn't commit to another dog. So the big new black dog rode down the hill with us in the back of the car and I kept turning around to look at him, to make sure he was real.

Now, there are two ways people have dogs out in the country where we live. You let them run, and hope they don't get hit. If you're lucky, you have dogs that stick close to home. Or you have an enclosure or a dog run, like people who have hunting dogs tend to do. Anyway, we did not have an enclosure and I would not risk losing another dog. So, we got a long line for him and, wonder of wonders, we let him come inside! I never thought Tim would let a dog inside, ever. He was a fan of barn animals with no inside fur and mess to deal with in the house. But there was something about this dog and the prospect of a companion for me that turned him around. The boys named him "Satchel" after a popular cartoon dog, and he became one of the family. There was one problem: he did not like kids. We knew he hadn't liked Dave's little girls but we thought that was because they were so little. He nipped at Jack and although I was convinced we had to get rid of him, Tim said we owed the dog a chance. We were his fourth owner and he had experienced a spotty upbringing.

There was a lot of damage to try to undo, but over the years we have learned how to deal with him and we have trained him to be good with us. I spent a lot of time just sitting next to him on his dog bed on the floor, waiting for him to look at me, or sniff me, and not reaching out to him until he was ready. My patience sealed the deal: he became, and still is, my devoted companion. Okay, we know Satchel can't go to social events with us, and he has to be contained if we have visitors, and he has nipped at one or two friends (I think they're still friends). Yet he has stayed so loyal and dedicated to me that I could never let him go now. He has been a healer in his own way. He stays by me and even now, when I walk him, he knows when to slow down and when to stop if I am having trouble keeping up with him.

During the months of May and June, Tim was busy readying the latest batch of songs for a new cd. I had co-written about half of the songs with him and was excited to see them come to fruition. He took me into the studio as soon as I could be without a mask, and we sang together. I was so grateful to be able to still sing, and to have input on the recording process. A song we had written a few months before I had been diagnosed—"Sometimes Trouble Is A Gift"—was particularly meaningful now. Another called "The Back Fields" was also poignant in light of the journey our family had been on for the past six months. It was important for Tim to have a project besides taking care of me, and a creative endeavor was sustaining for both of us. The cd "The Back Fields" was born that summer of recovery, and we released it with a concert in October, 2005.

I felt great. That summer was the gentlest and sweetest, in so many ways. Jack and Connor were considerate and helpful, constantly telling me to go sit in the hammock and read, or go lay down on the couch, what could they bring me? I floated from place to place, in the house or out in the fresh air. The dog, Satchel, stayed by my side and the boys would walk him so my arms wouldn't get tired. I was getting stronger every day. It was a concentrated time of healing and nurturing; I could feel it.

One morning, I remember it so well, I woke up and I felt "different". I couldn't identify exactly how different, but instead of wondering how I was going to get through the day, I felt as if I could get up and go. I told Tim he didn't have to drive me anywhere; I could do it myself. As I was driving around on some errands, I began to feel like ME. That was the thing; I felt like the "old" me, the one I remembered, the me I used to be. It was exhilarating. I saw the doctor that week and told him this. He said that was as important a part of his diagnosis as were the blood labs. Nobody knew how I should feel better than me; we all have the knowledge of our own wellness if we are paying attention to our bodies. My appetite had returned with a vengeance and I began to savor the tastes and textures of food once again. Ah, what a thrill.

MONDAY JUNE 20—I have been basically "kicked out of the nest" by Dr. Cripe. He says he only wants to see me once a month and that my treatment is finished. Now, it is just monitoring to make sure leukemia doesn't come back. I asked Dr. Cripe a question as he was finishing up with my paperwork. When I was in the hospital, there was one file that held all my various test results and daily vital signs and all the information on my condition; all the doctors could refer to that file, everyone knew where that file was and there was someone in charge. Now that I'm out on my own, I had to ask: Who's in charge?

He said that I was in charge of my own health. I said I didn't want to be! I was scared. He said that was a normal reaction, but that I really did need to be aware, to listen to my body, to be pro-active. But he said that overall, <u>he</u> was still in charge. I sighed in relief. I want him to be at the helm if anything should happen to me, because he could reference everything to leukemia. Oh, by the way, <u>my port is out</u>…let me say something about THAT!!! I got to take a shower for the first time since February 16. I have had a port in my chest or neck everyday since then and have been only able to take baths up to the neck. When I got in the shower, I almost couldn't get out…it was heaven. The weirdest part was not feeling the heaviness of my wet hair…because there was no hair…and my bald head got so cold when I got out. My hair is coming in a bit, kind of spotty like a dalmation. Aaah, the blessings of recovery. Love, Jan

So these were small but significant milestones. I began to think of leukemia as a bump in the road, a hurdle I had gotten over and I was now onto the rest of my life. I wondered if the website should be closed because there was really nothing more to report. I mean, who wanted to hear the minute details of my bodily functions? I didn't even want to write about them! So I proposed, in a journal entry, that perhaps it was time for our little community to close up shop. The response was an overwhelming "NO!" Almost everyone was in favor of keeping the website open. The people who wrote in all said how much it had meant for them to check in everyday, maybe not to write anything, but to see and hear what others were up to and to take solace in the sharing of so much hope and kindness. It had affected so many of us in ways we could never have foreseen. The web of interconnectedness was powerful.

My journal entries became fewer and farther between, because I was busy living, and there was no big news to report. It was confusing to know what to write, because I did not want to become a blogger who writes about her thoughts on any subject that comes to mind. There are enough blogs in the world and I didn't think my opinions were of that much consequence to anyone. I also didn't want to be looking for crises or dreadful events, just so I had something to write about.

MONDAY, JULY 4—An update on Independence Day: I am eating like a horse! And feeling good, although every tiny little ache or pain causes me to wonder, "is this leukemia?" I guess it will take me a while to accept the fact that I am well, and that life goes on. I still have the spots, which horrify my sons, and they have instructed me not to go out in public in shorts. Well, thank you very much, I wasn't planning to! Any other advice? -Jan

FRIDAY JULY 15—So much Real Life going on, I haven't had time to write! Connor turned thirteen last week and so we have the teenage thing going on in our house again. Fasten your seatbelts, parents; it's going to be a bumpy ride! Both boys go to camp next week and they are ready to go, even though we have all been thriving in so much togetherness. My sisters came to visit and entitled their trip "All About Jan". How cool is that? We went shopping, out to eat, to a museum; I even swam one night at their hotel, my first swim in what seemed like forever. I almost cried when I swam around underwater. I felt so light and so free. I did have an epiphany while shopping. I was trying on clothes and was seeing my body from every possible angle in those mirrored dressing rooms. I realized that the scrawny, saggy, spotted body in the mirror might have repulsed me, even a year ago, or at least would have elicited my pity. But now, that body looked fabulous to me. It was alive, most importantly, and it was ME and I'm in remission, and I think it's beautiful. What do you know? Love, Jan

There were little signs that I was progressing, and my radar was keenly attuned to any indication of progress. I was taking Satchel for longer walks and felt my stamina returning in increments. I also had enough hair, well "fuzz" is the more accurate word, to wash; I actually washed it with shampoo and rinsed it, and although it dried in about thirty seconds when I got out, it felt like hair; the beginnings of hair. I even taught a class for IRT, a distance learning class, of which I had done many in the years B.L. (before leukemia). This one was with students in Hong Kong! It was very exciting to be in front of the students again and even feel almost competent. I could answer questions off the cuff and I even came up with some witty comments. Little by little, I was getting back to my Life, just as we had planned long ago in the hospital on that cold February day.

When Tim and I got a call from the Indiana Repertory Theatre to perform in the first play of the season, "Inherit The Wind", we were feeling strong and I was ready to work. My part would not be too demanding, which was appropriate for my first time back to work. I was practically giddy the first day of rehearsal. The IRT has been our artistic home for some time now. And their care of me during my hospitalization was extraordinary. The nephew of the artistic director was struggling with cancer also, and they were all attuned to the vagaries of treatment and recovery. They were equally jubilant to bring me back to work. It was like coming home.

During this time, my friends in Chicago organized a benefit concert for us to help with our medical bills, which were accumulating in piles and piles of paper in our office. Rita, Janet, Lois, Denise, and Jan all worked together to make it an extravaganza with amazing food, while Dave and his band provided music. I felt vulnerable as I got up to the microphone that night to thank everyone. I was practically bald still (just the spotted fuzz) and so many people had shown up, including old friends, fans of Tim's music, Lucas and a group of his college friends, and on and on. It was an outpouring of love and support. I felt grateful, and also odd to up on stage because I had been sick. I have since come to understand that people want to help, they want to contribute in any way they can, because otherwise they feel helpless. So it isn't about me being the center of attention as much as it is about letting people help. That's not always easy to do. I am still learning about that.

It was fun to be back at work and I was also writing a play for middle school audiences about kids moving to Indiana from other countries. The influx of immigrants has really impacted the Indiana schools and there are finally starting to be significant efforts to help in that transition. Understanding on all sides of the issue is the goal.

It was so affirming to be working. When I was sick, both in and out of the hospital, I felt like I had lost some part of my identity. To be thinking and working and conversing with smart adults and collaborating creatively was validating and nurturing. I felt stronger everyday. Tim had composed and was performing the music for the play "Inherit The Wind" and we were having a blast working together. It was also wonderful to be in a dressing room again with other women. Jolene, Kate, and Mattie were all excited about my recovery. We talked about the illness a lot in the dressing room. It is curious because it seems most people are uncomfortable with talking about cancer, even though they're anxious to know what it's like, or how it happened—all the details. I had no compunction about relaying my stories, because I thought they were pretty fascinating also! Not that I am particularly fascinating. It's the illness and the stories around it that are compelling. In any case, I didn't mind talking about it at all, and sometimes we found ourselves laughing hysterically at some nutty detail of some hospital story and when we'd sober up, one of us would say, "I can't believe we're laughing about leukemia!!" and that would crack us up all over again.

It was so gratifying to be back on stage again. I love that theatre especially; the IRT is a big house but an intimate one, and it is a beautifully restored piece of antiquity. As a cast, we were all friendly and respectful of each other, which is always a treat. Our director, Michael, was a gracious and lovely man and one time when we had all gone out to eat on a dinner break during our tech rehearsals, he remarked to me with characteristic flair, "Darling, you look wonderful." And I said, "Well thank-you, I feel wonderful." And he said, "Isn't it absolutely a miracle what you've been through? You know? It has made us all better people. We were never so alive as when you were sick." Whoa. That was a big statement to make, and I realized it was true. It was true in some ways for me too. The closer to death we are, the more alive we feel, if we're lucky enough to be aware of it, or at least to be able to see it that way. Sometimes trouble is a gift.

The most wonderful thing happened for me after the play opened. I began to rehearse for the next play at IRT: "A Christmas Carol"!! I had wanted to do this play for years; almost every actor I know has done a part of some sort in a production of this play somewhere. I never had the time, or the ability to make that commitment at the holiday when the kids were little, and I was over the moon to finally get to do it. I was cast as "Sister of Mercy" and the "Char-Woman" as well as some other dancing and singing parts. In the IRT production, nobody rests…you are on stage most of the time and it is hard, physical work. But so gratifying. I heard Dickens' words over and over and they only became more and more meaningful and beautiful as the rehearsals continued. Again, I was in a dressing room full of funny and smart women and we talked about everything, with cancer now taking a back seat in the conversations. There were many more pressing matters to discuss, like our kids and our husbands and fashion and gossip. Just the normal fare of the dressing room, and it was great to be back to normal.

The "Christmas Carol" cast is a group of actors that rotates and changes slightly from year to year. In this particular cast, I was one of two new people. Everyone else had previous experience with this production, so there was a kind of shorthand in the staging of the play. Everyone except us two "newbies" knew what the hell they were doing, and how the set was going to be transformed into the many different scenes that we would be creating. For example, we were in a scene that didn't have real doors, but we were supposed to look as if we coming through doors. But that wasn't clear to me, so when our director, Priscilla, said, "Okay, now, you're all going to answer the doors." I said, "What doors?" Well, for some reason, that absolutely undid everyone. Even still, just the words "What doors?" make those who were there fall apart laughing. It was one of many mishaps for me as I learned the show, and it became a running joke that I was recovering from leukemia. If I misunderstood something, or went to the wrong place on stage, I'd say, "Hey, I'm in remission!" It was our running joke…she's in remission. Everybody wanted to be "in remission"—it was such a great excuse.

As I look back at all the journal and guestbook entries from the website, and my own personal journal and notes from that time, I see there were very few entries. I was working and living and I was not sick. The website seemed like a thing for sick people and that wasn't me anymore. My last two journal entries were the following:

SEPTEMBER 2—I was at IU Med Center for some routine tests and I was early, so I decided to go up and see if any of the nurses I knew on 5-N were there. It was so completely strange to be there, to know where to go, to have that familiarity with the place. I remembered the last time I was there, I had been masked, gloved, and gowned and running up and down the halls, not caring what anybody thought. So it was a different story to be there as a well person. At first, nobody recognized me. I am 15 pounds heavier and I have hair! It was so great to see them, especially Mary H., who had seen me through many dark times. They are all still there, taking care of the next sick person that comes in, never ceasing in their work, their caring, their professionalism. I have driven by the hospital many times since I was there, and I think: they're all in there, working away. Who knew how lucky we were to have such people doing that job? Who knew that IU Med Center was so fabulous, that right here in the cornfields was one of the best places to go for treatment of leukemia? I didn't have to travel to another city, to a big cancer center. There was one in my back yard.

OCTOBER 12—Hi all. I am writing what I think is the last journal entry for a while. At least I don't have any plans to write for a long time. This website will stay open for people to communicate, wrap things up, and get e-mail addresses for each other. I am living in a state of wellness and health and I am just getting on with my life, loving my husband and children, and writing and acting, trying to keep the kitchen floor clean and the lawn mowed. Oh man, mundane life is so sweet. The leukemia seems like a dream…almost like something that happened to somebody else. But when I read the journal or talk to my friends who were in the hospital with me, I know it did happen. Sometimes I still get scared with the "what-ifs" about the future and the possibility of relapse. But if I remember to close my eyes and breathe and feel the health I now possess, I am comforted and swept back into Real Life in the Now. It's been one of the hardest and most valuable lessons: staying in the moment. Worrying does not take care of tomorrow, it robs today of it joy. I think about leukemia every day and I wonder about it and how some people get cancer and some people don't and how it is such a teacher and destroyer at the same time. I know my life will never be the same. I am in awe of the love that was sent to me by all of you and I thank everyone for the words, head scarves, pajamas, donations to our medical account, DVDs and cds and books and lotions and teas and fuzzy blankets and special pillows and photos and drawings and meditation aids and yoga tapes and socks and slippers and meals to our home, for healing prayers and vibes and for every second of time that you ever spent thinking about me…it has all carried me to where I am and that is alive. Very alive! Peace. Thank-you. Love, Jan P.S. I am still drawing and writing a lot about the journey…who knows what that will become?

7

The IRT production of "A Christmas Carol" has a unique set. It is a large open stage covered with snow. Of course, it's "stage snow", fake stuff made from shredded plastic milk bottles or something like that. None of the actors really know what it is, but we all had stories about it coming home in our shoes or underwear. Actors who had done the show many times before spoke of finding it somewhere in their house or in their clothes in the summertime. The stuff is everywhere! It is designed to cover a number of props which emerge and then hide again after they've been used. But navigating around those props is a challenge. I asked, during rehearsal, how do you know where things are? The answer was mystical: "you just know…" Okay, I guessed I'd find out. The first day on the stage in what is called "Tech rehearsal" I was dressed in my huge Victorian gown with a heavy cloak over it to enter through the house (the audience) singing and up onto the stage for the opening song of the second act. I was the last in line and was hurrying to get to my place, when BOOM! I tripped over a large frame that is hidden under the snow and went flying. Everyone was worried because, as they knew only too well, I was in remission! There was a hush and when they saw I was laughing, they all began to laugh. It was the first of the many physical rigors I would experience doing the show. I also had to come up onto the stage through a trap door. As the "Char Woman", I was laden with heavy skirts and shawls and a bag slung over my shoulder. Getting the timing of that opening and the strength to heave it and the bag out on stage required all my efforts. Once I got it, I had no problems. There was a great deal of dancing as well. I was lucky to be partnered with my friend and fellow actor David, who had much experience with the show, and could move me handily around the stage, leaping and spinning and twirling all the way. During rehearsals, he used to say, "Alright, who's got Jan?" He was referring to the fact that when I didn't know where to go next, he (or someone) was always telling me in a loud whisper, "Go stage left! Or head upstage to the lantern!" Everyone was taking care of me because…you guessed it: I was in remission!

So the whole process was taxing but exhilarating. We did two weeks of student matinees before we were to open for the public. I had a moment in the show when I was a "snowbird", as one of the narrator parts was called, and I would sit on the stage and watch the actor playing Scrooge look out into the audience as if he could see his own childhood, and he would say in awe, "I was bred in this place…" Every single time, I was moved to tears by that scene. It was deeply emotional and deeply psychological. Today we speak of going back to our childhood to learn about our present self and about how our ability to handle situations is formed by our youth…Dickens knew all that and more. His character, Scrooge, has the ultimate journey of forgiveness and redemption. It is a magnificent story and I understood it in a deeper way than ever before. I absolutely LOVED doing that play! Also, there was something about the material that brought out the best in the whole cast, which was a very good thing. There are all kinds of attitudes and difficulties that can arise when dealing with a large cast doing such a rigorous piece. But our group got along well, and there was also a good deal of kindness for the six child actors who took turns playing the children's roles. One of the actresses and I used to lay back on the cool floor in our giant dresses before we went on at a certain part, and we'd whisper back stage and share stories about our children and our lives. She was the first person that I told about the deep aches and pains that were starting to come with regularity in my chest, ribs and neck. I was afraid of what it might mean and she was a compassionate listener. She reminded me of Carol, who had kept repeating that first night of diagnosis. "Well, we don't know what it is, so we can't worry yet…" Grace said much the same. "Don't worry yet, it might just be the strain of the show itself."

I went for my regular check-up at the Hematology Clinic one Monday, which was our day off, and I explained my symptoms. I had an uncomfortable feeling of pressure when I would take a deep breath, like I couldn't open up my lungs all the way, and it hurt. Blood tests revealed the presence of "blasts" and Dr. Cripe said it was the beginning of a relapse.

Relapse?

Relapse.

That <u>word</u>. It was a black hole that I seemed to be falling into. The room started spinning and the doctor and his nurse looked like they were receding into space. "Jan!" I blinked and shook my head. "Relapse? RELAPSE??" He nodded. I sort of crumpled in the chair. "No. No. No." was all I could say. This could NOT be happening. I had done everything right, I had done everything I was supposed to do, I had fought the fight like a good soldier-patient and I was supposed to be well. <u>That</u> was how it was supposed to be. I am sure I cried at this point; I don't even remember what happened next. My memories of this time are very sketchy. I know Dr. Cripe and Sheryl pulled their chairs up close to mine but I don't remember what we said or how I got home or how I told Tim. Dr. Cripe did say that I could continue to do the show as long as I felt like I could, but that we would begin the process for a Bone Marrow Transplant now. There would be no second attempt at chemo since I had not stayed in remission very long

I had to tell the theatre administration that there was a possibility that I could not finish the run of the show and that they needed to get a replacement lined up. We were lucky that many people who had done the show before worked at the theatre, and so my friend and colleague, Milicent, turned out to be the one who would be "on deck" if it should come to that. I told the girls in my dressing room also since we had all told each other everything, and I didn't want them to be surprised if I did have to leave.

It was difficult to continue on with life, with the show, with motherhood, driving around as usual but knowing that something was growing in my bones again, and that something was leukemia. It was like carrying around a lead weight in my chest. That was where the pain was most noticeable, in my chest, especially when I would take a deep breath. I felt the weight of my costume and the effort of dancing getting more and more burdensome. The joke about me being in remission wasn't funny anymore, but only a few of us knew that. I didn't want to tell everyone and have them worried and over-careful with me on stage. I wanted things to be as normal as possible.

We did tell our boys that I was not in remission anymore and that I was going to have to go back in the hospital at some point but we didn't know when. They were both incredulous; how could this be happening? But they carried on, probably keeping their worry inside for they had been through it before.

Opening night of "A Christmas Carol" for the public was thrilling because we finally had adults in the audience. My family was there, and Liz's family, and I felt like I was giving them a gift. This show had come to mean so much to me, and I loved doing it for people I loved. The next day I came in to do the second evening show, and when it came to the part where I was under the stage, and had to pop open the trap door and fling myself out as the Char Woman, I couldn't do it. I got the door open about halfway, and almost cried out—I just didn't have the strength. The other actors were watching me, anticipating my entrance, and when I couldn't get out in the usual amount of time, their eyes widened in worry. Finally, I gave one last heave, and the door slammed open. I hauled myself up on the stage and we finished the scene. By the end of the show, I was in tears. I knew I couldn't go on. We called Janet, the artistic director, to the dressing room and I fell apart. There was a pall over the dressing room area as everyone found out the news: I had relapsed.

I felt like such a failure. It is absurd, of course, to feel like you've "failed" because the disease isn't concerned with success or failure. But I had worked SO hard at getting well, I had worked SO hard at being a good patient and doing everything I was supposed to do. I had educated myself, I had learned the lingo, I had given myself injections, and ingested hundreds of pills. We had paid thousands of dollars in co-payments for medications and services and insurance premiums, we had waded through stacks of paperwork. It seemed impossible. I couldn't completely comprehend it, but I knew it was happening in my body because I was losing energy and strength and willpower.

I didn't go back to the show after that night. It seemed ridiculous to even try to get through it, feeling so lousy. Milicent went on the next night with a script in her hand, eventually memorized my part, and finished the run of the show. I called Dr. Cripe and said "Okay, let's get this ball rolling. I'm done with the show, I want to get this chemo over with." I grabbed my drawing paper one day and scribbled the picture "Relapse" in about five minutes. It felt good to express my anger that way. Then I wrote in the website journal:

> NOVEMBER 30—I will go back to IU Med Center tomorrow and begin the prep for the chemo to be administered in exactly the same way that I had it before last Feb. I will be in the hospital for 28-30 days, then home to recover. Then, in about a month and a half, back in for a bone marrow transplant, which will entail five days of more intensive chemo (I can't even imagine such a thing) and then an infusion of new blood cells and then 20 or so days of waiting to see if my body rejects them, or if they reject me! Quite a grueling prospect, but I am determined to get through it and live the rest of my days! I still have so much to do: books and plays to write and pictures to draw and kids to watch grow up and I am definitely not ready to check out just yet. More news later when we get more details.

I walked into the hospital on December 1st and I was not a happy person. I couldn't even fake it. Tim and I rode the elevator up to 5-N. I went down that familiar hallway, turned into my little room, and sat on the bed and cried. There was the Blue Chair and there was the window with the slatted blind, and there was the bed and the curtain, all plain, all too familiar, and all sickening. My first few days were grim. I went through the usual: got the port put in my neck, got all the vitals taken, got all the meds, started the chemo. I was in a dark mood. This time, I did not want ANY visitors and I was cranky and grumpy. I drew a picture of a half-naked girl on a burning bed, with the words on the bottom "What chemo??"

One day my friend Carla came to give me a massage and brought with her another masseuse, Frieda, who is also a "healer" of sorts. Frieda had a wise and peaceful countenance, and when they entered and asked if they could do some "energy work" with me, I said, "Fine. Why not." After the women had touched me and lightly massaged my legs and back and feet, Frieda said, "Jan, you're so angry. You have to make friends with this chemo if that's your choice of medical path, because if you don't, you're fighting it the whole way. Your body needs the energy to withstand the chemo and let it do its job. You have to find ways to sustain yourself through this."

Harummpph! is what I thought of that. I smiled wanly and nodded, saying good-bye, anxious for them to get out of my room. After they left, I sat there alone with my thoughts, once again. I started to have that feeling…the one when you know someone is right, even though you don't want them to be. Oh damn. She was right; I did have to make a commitment to this path, I had to embrace the cure even though it was painful. Again.

That was one big step towards making this hospital stay more bearable. The next step happened when a woman who had received a bone marrow transplant two years ago came to visit me, at my doctor's request. She was not especially remarkable at first glance. She came from a small town somewhere in eastern Indiana, she was a few years older than me, wanted to live to see her grandkids grow, and she told me it had been hard, but she did it. There it was: she just did it. If she could do it, so could I. I felt the tide turning inside of me as I grasped the enormity of the task ahead. But with the cheers coming in waves from the sidelines, how could I not fight? Every last person who found out I had relapsed must have told ten people because the news hit the Internet and messages were once again pouring in. "You can do this" "We're with you!" "We're praying/singing/meditating/sending vibes"—you name it, they were doing it!

So I wrote a journal entry before I would be too sick to do so. I didn't want to kvetch too much but I also wanted to be honest about how "sucky", in fact, it was.

Dec. 3—Well, I've been in my "hotel room" as Tim calls it (room service and everything) for three days. The chemo started Thursday night and it is comprised of three different chemicals, each of which runs an hour each in succession. They are fondly referred to as "mec" which stands for Mitoxantrone, Etoposide (VP-16) and Cytosar (ARA-C) Plus a gazillion other meds coming in through the port in my neck and pills to be swallowed…I am a walking pharmacopoeia! I am slightly nauseated but less achy than I was two days ago. The aches in my bones were actually from the "blasts" overpacking my bones and that is being dealt with handily. I have been told to expect different side effects and I am thinking "worse"…sorry, the realist in me has taken over. I do not feel like the mighty warrior of last February. I am resolved to get through this and will do what is asked of me and get my body back to health. But I am not so cheerful or upbeat in my heart of hearts. I am so disheartened to be here again, so weary of the fight ahead, and so disappointed that all the work we ALL did together doesn't seem to have been enough. What is the universe telling me? Phoooey. -Jan

In spite of my foul attitude, I began to decorate my room. I mean, you just have to; you have to take the hospital scene and adjust it slightly to be your own experience; your own icons or reminders of your life have to imbue the room with your essence. The things that locate a person in the world are so unavailable in an extreme hospital situation, and bringing pieces of your outside life in really helps remind you of who you are. Our friend Jane brought a hammered metal sculpture to hang on the wall called "Tree Of Life". I could stare at it for many minutes at a time, it seemed so hopeful. Janet came with Hannukah lights and Pris brought an angel for above the bed. Then a very wonderful decoration arrived: Amie had brought a little plastic tree with lights and tiny ornaments and…tiny black and white pictures of my family. Here was Jack putting a hat on Buddy, our spotted horse. Here was Connor, looking goofy at the camera. There was Tim, playing guitar in our living room. There was Lucas smiling on our front porch, and there was me! In the old days, but still me on the inside. I could look at all the pictures with the lights twinkling all around, and I felt a little less depressed.

DECEMBER 5—This is Julie, hating that Jan's not up to writing, so it's me again until she gets better. Yesterday was rough. She's getting the big chemo cocktail and she's very nauseated. Her appetite is gone, her port is itchy, she's getting a fever and rashes, and aches and pains need to be dulled by various meds. She's strong though, still laughing and focused on tomorrow. She had gotten so strong during her remission so seemed healthier to go back in. Her nurses are her old friends from before and are taking good care of her. Jan meets the BMT doctor today to learn the details of what's ahead. This is yet a new chapter.

I did meet the doctor that day. I was told to have two people with me to hear the whole scoop, with one person writing it all down, and all of us listening to see if we all heard the same thing. So I picked one of my most intellectual friends, Janet, who would be a stickler for details and knew something about cancer treatment already from her nephew's battle up in Chicago. She knew the lingo. And of course, I had my friend Liz, because she would listen with her heart and she is fearless about asking questions. So I awaited Dr. Robert Nelson with some trepidation. I was not anxious to be turned over to another doctor after I had grown so close to Dr. Cripe. But it was made very clear that a transplant was a different thing altogether than the standard chemo treatment for leukemia. Dr. Cripe had recommended Dr. Nelson to be my doctor.

Tim and I had been given lots of advice about what cancer centers and/or transplant centers I might consider for the upcoming phase of treatment. I had looked into a few of them, and all of them would have meant moving to another location for the duration of the transplant. Tim asked Dr. Cripe what would he do if his wife was facing a transplant, and he said wisely, "Well, I'd let my wife decide for herself, of course, with input from me if she asked. But if it was me, I'd go with Bob Nelson." Say no more.

So I was lying in bed, and my two friends had their pens and paper out and in walked Dr. Nelson. I remember my first impression so well. He was tall, and very serious, and wore a crisp white shirt, a dark tie, black pants and black shoes. This, after Dr. Cripe's wild flowery ties and Birkenstock shoes! I tried to listen to his thorough and complicated explanation of the transplant process but I was gradually losing focus and I hoped my friends were getting it all. My teeth began to chatter, and I sank down into my blankets. Dr. Nelson looked over at me, shot up and said, "This patient is sick. She has a fever!" He buzzed for the nurse, got my temperature, checked my antibiotics and got me on Tylenol right away. He tucked the blankets around me, helped me drink a sip of water, and then resumed his discussion of the transplant with Janet and Liz while I slept. The next day, he came back to see me. He said we would go over it again, and again, and probably again, so that he was sure I understood what was going to happen. There was something so honest about Dr. Nelson, and so thoughtful. I felt like I could trust him. The journey toward transplant had begun.

> Dec. 11—Greetings from snowy Indiana! This is Liz again as Jan isn't up to writing. She has had a couple of good days however, and sends her greetings and love to everyone. When I arrived yesterday a.m. she was taking a jaunt around the ward with her BMT doc. Dr. Nelson, who very thoughtfully came by to see her and reassure her that he was taking care of her from afar at this point. He said he was getting very familiar with her case and thinking about her a lot. Nice guy. They were yukking it up in the hallway and then I practically had to jog to keep up with her back to her room on 5-N! We had a nice visit and then she fell asleep. She has been sleeping better which does a lot for her spirits. Her friend Lee came down from Chicago and spent the night with her and Jan really enjoyed that. The process for finding a match for her blood profile has begun. By the way, many people have asked about having their blood tested to see if they could donate to Jan. She wants to encourage everyone to go into the bone marrow registry but you are not able to designate who gets your cells. If you want info about the registry, go to www.marrow.org. This is a great website, full of information. -Liz

I did another drawing during this time of a pile of clothes scattered about a hospital room and a body floating high above. I titled it,

"All that Was Left Were Her Clothes". My drawings during this time were dark and brooding. Relapse was just an air-sucking, life-deflating, depressing word. I was going through the motions of my regular demeanor, but underneath I was so depressed. Why me? This question haunted me. Why? How does this happen to people? I know there is cause and effect so what's the cause of this genetic anomaly that makes my bone marrow malfunction? It seemed that there must be a mystery deep within a mystery about sickness and healing and our medical techniques have just scratched the surface

I had a total meltdown one morning as I was putting on shoes and socks and getting ready to go on a walk with Tim in the hallway. I was frozen, mid-sock, feeling Tim's eyes on me and unable to look up at his beautiful warm face…what if I never see it again? I am not ready to leave him. I don't want to be disabled or disfigured from all of this…what if the transplant messes up my body? I'll be alive, but not me, not the Jan that Tim married. Sadness was so big in my heart right then. I didn't want to voice my thoughts for fear of ruining the morning.

Another morning as I walked the halls, the absurdity (or was it the reality?) of it all hit me: I have leukemia and I'm in my own world with my own drama in this hospital. I can hear TV's in rooms and people talking and the ever-present beep of someone's machine somewhere. "I do not want this illness." I may have said it out loud. I wanted to be well, to live my life. I was so profoundly sad at that moment, trapped in this diseased body, trapped by leukemia, weighed down by my own sadness. I missed my boys. I missed my dog. I wanted to run out of there and walk out in our woods and soak up Mother Earth, up into my bones and blood, and heal. It occurred to me that I could leave. Just leave and go home.

Dr. Cripe had told me that going through the bone marrow transplant was a choice, an active choice, not something you let happen to you. Well, great. I mulled this over, finally arriving at the thought: what other choice did I have? I suppose I could go home and slowly decline, and not go through the harrowing difficulties and risks of transplant. But I wanted more Life. More Life! That became my inner mantra. So I hunkered down in my room, knitting (badly) and watching bad TV, just trying not to be there, not to think, just to distract myself. It looked like I'd probably be in the hospital for Christmas, and that was a low blow. The boys would have to wrap their heads around that concept.

Oh yes, I was pretty depressed. Even my little room, which had come to look like a beautiful nook—filled with pictures and holiday lights strung all over, a little fake tree decorated with tiny photos of my family—none of this could cheer me up. I was stuck deep inside my sadness. I had also been sicker than before so that took its toll. I had been experiencing what they called "rigors" or extreme chills, despite the fact that I had no fever. Finally, I was given broad-spectrum antibiotics and painkillers and I began to feel better. One day, a teddy bear arrived in a box with an anonymous note that read, "Here's a bear you can tell all your troubles to." It was odd, but that bear felt so comforting, like there was someone else in the room with me. I loved the fact that the sender remained mysterious and I have that bear still, sitting in a place of authority in my office. I was extremely fortunate to have a network of loving support, but still, there I was, going through cancer treatment. No one could do it for me. Aloneness, in the most profound way.

I got the Big News that a donor had been found. She was a 33-year-old woman who had never had children, which is a good thing because of the antibodies that are found in women who have been pregnant. I couldn't know anything else about the donor until a year has passed after the transplant; she would remain anonymous to me until then. A few hurdles remained: she had to have a physical and her blood had to pass some tests, so they were searching for a back-up just in case. This promise of a donor perked us all up and we focused on what was to come. On December 23, I was told that I could go home the next day, Christmas Eve. I would be home for Christmas; I couldn't believe it. Yes!

The day of the 24th, I woke up early and started to pack up all my things. I went from passively accepting that I would have to be in the hospital for what seemed like forever, to needing to get out NOW. I packed, dressed, sat on my bed and waited for doctors' rounds. I could not eat the breakfast that was brought; I honestly thought I could not eat one single bite more of hospital food. It turned out to be a long day, because I needed platelets and a red blood transfusion before I could go home. At five o'clock, Tim and I drove out of the hospital parking garage and headed home. I arrived on Christmas Eve to a decorated living room, a tree all lit up, a fire in the fireplace, and two boys oohing and aahing over all the presents. The angels of Columbus and Chicago, namely Suzanne and Rita, had done the Christmas shopping for us (I don't think the boys will ever again see such loot!)

There was a bittersweet quality to that week. I had been so cautioned and apprised of the danger facing me regarding the transplant, that I couldn't help but wonder if this was my last Christmas. That was the reality of the situation, because the chemo before a transplant is so much more intense than what I had gone through before, in order to take the bone marrow down to nothing, the effects of that regimen on my organs that would most likely be the cause of any fatality. Tim and I knew this; we had spoken the words "death" and "dying". Dr. Cripe had explained the process to all of us—Lucas, Connor and Jack all came to my room with Tim, and Dr. Cripe told of the dangers of the extreme chemo, adding, "I would be remiss if I didn't tell you that your mom could die from this." We were all somber after that meeting. Jack climbed into bed with me and I put my arms around him and reassured them that I was NOT planning on that course of action and I would be alive for many years still to hound them about their messy rooms and homework. Tim and Lucas looked at each other and stayed quiet. The memory of Dr. Cripe's words hung in the air and floated around on the back of all our minds, whether we were aware of it or not.

So every moment at home was a precious one. I would look around at everyone and have this secret longing to just wrap them in my arms and stay that way forever. But of course, you don't do that, especially not with adolescent boys. But I was allowed to be a little more "huggy" than usual and I took full advantage of it.

My illness had taken on a mystical quality. It had a transformative power once again and it was like being under a spell. Part of it was the waiting period, like a kind of limbo, a kind of dream. I was so whittled down, pared down to the essence of me, and experiencing my family around me as I was in that state was oddly satisfying. It was as if I was in the presence of something holy, walking a line between life and death. I would lie on that couch and watch them all coming and going, just being themselves, and I felt as if I could see beyond that, beyond their humanness. It was profound and I felt like I had a secret. I guess I did.

My dog Satchel (that grumpy one) shunned me for the first day home. He had sniffed me and apparently smelled something foreign and not to his liking. I had to patiently wait, talking to him gently, before he realized that it was <u>me</u>, his companion and newfound friend. After that, he sat by my side as I lay on the couch and wouldn't move. He viewed anyone who came close to me with suspicion. He was keeping vigil.

DEC. 28—Hi Folks. Tim here. I'm writing in Jan's stead as we begin to meet the calm after Christmas. The tree was trimmed, the kitchen newly painted golden yellow with red trim (thanks Dad and Aunt Janeo) and Jan arrived home to all her "men" on Christmas Eve. Much generosity from family and friends for the boys under the tree but the real gift was just having Jan home. She has made herself a cozy spot on the couch where she can sleep, watch the fire and revel in Satchel's attention. The days are generally good but she is a bit nauseated still and tires easily. Tonight she feels depleted and may need a transfusion tomorrow. We're waiting…have our first real appointment with the bone marrow doctor, Dr. Nelson, after the first of the year. Trying to build up strength for the long haul. Keep writing, sending your vibes and jokes and memories and LOVE. Best, Tim

Enlightenment seemed to come in fits and starts. I had probably heard the various pieces of information about my leukemia and the treatment in different ways each time they were explained to me. When I was home, ruminating on the information about my upcoming transplant and spinning it around in my mind, it made for a cloudy picture. Time seemed to be stretching out and slowing down. It seemed as if I was languishing, not doing anything to get on with the transplant. So I went to the next doctor appointment with some "piss and vinegar". I may have even stamped my foot. "What's holding this up? Let's get this bone marrow transplant underway! Come ON, I'm home from the hospital and I'm just hanging there, waiting, waiting, waiting for someone to call, or something to happen…don't we have to get this thing underway before I relapse?" I was on fire, not my usual good-natured and agreeable patient-self. I was always a good listener, asking questions dutifully and digesting information before I reacted. This day was different. Dr. Cripe was very patient with me and re-described the process. He said we were not in a race to get this done. If I was going to relapse that fast, I'd probably do it even with the transplant. Also, there were many factors regarding my own health, which would need to be resolved before I would be in good enough shape to undergo the transplant…number one being the spot of pneumonia that still lingered, and the mouth and gum sores which continued to plague me. He said I had to be in optimum health to withstand the chemo and that could take some time. So the upshot was that it's a big balancing act, a dance of sorts, to get everything lined up for the procedure. And it's a matter of timing with the donor as well. I had a CT scan to verify the lung situation and another scan to check out my heart (wanting it to be found strong again, physically and poetically, like before). Many steps to take before climbing the mountain. The result of all this sturm and drang is that I felt comforted just by KNOWING. I could handle more information and I was at peace with the enormity of it all. Tim and my sister Pat both suggested that I bide my time this month with lots of movies and manicures, maybe even a pedicure! I finally came to the realization that this time was a gift. I had to ask myself: when else would I have Time without obligations? No volunteering, no work, no teaching, no enchiladas for the basketball team…no nothing! Except Time.

I finally went in for my BMT appointment with Dr. Nelson. There were still some unknowns but we were getting closer to answers. I had a bone marrow biopsy and the results would be key: if I was not in remission, we would go to Plan Z, whatever that was…I didn't exactly know. But if I was in remission, the doctors were considering a different version of the transplant, called the non-myoablative, or the "mini". This means the chemotherapy before the transplant is not as radical, does not wipe out the entire bone marrow, and would be much less harrowing to go through. There are pros and cons to this but it seemed mostly pros. The fatality rate for the "mini" is much less than for the conventional transplant, yet the question remains: is it as effective in ridding the body of leukemia and keeping it away? Doctor Nelson was fabulous: smart, clear, thoughtful and very trust inspiring. I felt so amazingly blessed to have both Dr. Cripe and Dr. Nelson so close to home at IU Med Center I have heard some discouraging stories about people's experiences with their doctors- the doctors don't listen to them or they are unpleasant or dismissive. But I have not had one single experience like that or any situation where I received less than the best care. Lucky me. The following week, I would get the Big Work-Up to see if I was all there to go in for the BMT.

JANUARY 24—We're honing in on a date! Looks like I'll be admitted on Feb. 7. I will have seven days of chemo and receive the new cells on the 14th. (I entered the hospital with my initial diagnosis on the 16th of Feb. one year ago...what a year!) The results of my tests were good and the donor passed her physical, so all signs say, "GO". So here's how we talk about it: the days before the transplant are referred to in "minus terms". In other words, the day I enter will be called Day -7. It goes on with Day -6, Day -5 etc. until Day 0, which is the transplant itself. Then every day after that is called "plus", like Day +1, Day +2. Sort of like a new life. I will have a new immune system and a new blood type, and then I will just live my life from then on! There are a wide variety of complications that happen post-transplant, but I know of so many success stories and I am planning on being one of those. It's so wild to be in this pre-adventure time. I am finally doing what I said I'd do and that is to just enjoy the TIME that I have. It is like time is standing still and every single thing is just so intensely beautiful and pleasing: the bare trees, the frozen puddles on the lane, my boys, the dog, the air, the stars at night, even Jack grumbling about being woken up in the morning doesn't irritate me, just makes me smile. The teen-agers are acting the way they're supposed to, the days are just unfolding the way they're supposed to and nobody can really say what each day will bring…they just roll on and on. There are so many people and everyone is trying to get through this life and then there's leukemia? It just is. Well, I wax philosophical here…it's a side effect of the situation. Back to sweeping the kitchen floor and walking the dog…it's all part of the same thing. All the energy that comes from my friends and family and even mere acquaintances who send best wishes—all conspires to help me get well and live—that's what I want: more of this crazy, unpredictable, fabulous Life. Thank you, Jan

FEBRUARY 4—I received the most amazing message on the machine yesterday: it was the Bone Marrow Transplant Coordinator, Jay, saying we are on schedule for admission on the 7th; in fact he had the travel itinerary for the cells…they will arrive the evening of the fourteenth! Miraculous news: my cells are coming. It's better than Christmas. Such a gift coming from…somewhere. I think of my donor everyday and pray for her health and well-being and hope my gratitude flies through the air right into her heart. I can't wait to meet her. Connor says I should spend the whole summer lying in the hammock and reading. He is so smart, that boy. I've been up at IU Med Center a lot lately. I had my lung capacity tested. That was interesting. I had to let all the air out of my lungs, as much, and then more, as I thought I could. Then I had to steadily take in air and keep on going until I thought I would burst. My lungs were good; not great, but good. The technicians who were operating the measuring device commented on my yellow shirt and lavender sweater. They said how lovely the colors were, but that they could never wear such bright colors. I thought to myself, "You never know what you can do till you have leukemia!" Anyone can wear bright colors. You just need to not be afraid.

My insurance company assigned me a case manager and she informed me, with a trace of ice in her voice, that I needed a colonoscopy, a pap smear, a dental exam, a mammogram, and a psychological evaluation before I could go into the hospital. All this 12 days before admission date. Well, it all was accomplished and faxed in and when I was up seeing all the docs, they said I was the healthiest-looking sick woman they'd ever seen! Dr. Nelson said I looked bright and chipper, something I haven't heard since my mom called me that at age 15. He said it's a great time for a transplant.

He knows these things. -Jan

So I was waiting for the Big Day and just "being". Tim and I decided I should go with him on a four-day music tour out East. I don't usually go with him because the boys' schedules are pretty demanding and asking someone to take care of all that is a big request. But we love to go on the road together, and in light of the upcoming ordeal, I thought I should just do it. It took extensive planning, but once we headed out on the highway, I knew I had done the right thing. We played music in Syracuse, then on to Bradford, Vermont and then to do a "house concert" on our way home.

A house concert is a phenomenon unique to folk music. They come in different shapes and sizes, but the basics are the same: a person opens their house to guests and an invited musician(s) comes to play for them. It can be a small living room with 14 people, or it can be a backyard with 60 people. There are all kinds of ways to get people into a house and we've seen a lot of them. The audience can fill someone's large basement or be crowded into a study attached to a dining room, with people sitting on the stairs and out in the front hall. A house concert host may have a mailing list and charge admission, or he/she might invite select friends and pass the hat. In any format, it is most always a delight for the musician, because the people really want to be there. They are usually music lovers and the goal is a common one: to have a great time, to have fun, to gather together with music.

I think folk music could save the world, if there were enough of these house concerts, partially for the fact that musicians often stay the night with the hosts or are put up by a guest of the concert. When Tim goes on the road, even when he's playing at a club or concert series, he often stays with people who host the musicians when they come through town. This does a couple of things: it lets him into people's houses, and gives him a window into how other people live, which is enlightening and instructive. Also, he shares his experiences as an actor and musician and can educate people about what it is really like to make a living as an artist. So it's a very fruitful two-way street, and understanding grows on both sides of the relationship. I'm always amazed at Tim's ability to be at ease with complete strangers and how they are not strangers by the time he leaves. I'm also surprised and gratified by the hospitality people are willing to show to a traveling musician. For such a talkative person as myself, I am surprisingly shy in these situations, but I love just being on the road with Tim.

This trip proved to be delightful as always. Just getting in the car together and driving is a treat for us. We each point out interesting sights to the other: a round barn, a group of steamy black cows huddled in the snow, a hand painted sign proclaiming "HAY", a small weathered blue shack that says "Anne's Autos". One sign we remember from out west read: "Dogs Worrying Or Harming The Livestock May Be Shot". Hmm, you don't see that very often.

On this trip we held the knowledge in our hearts of the upcoming transplant, which could and probably would change our lives forever. There was a quiet intensity to the trip, as well as unabashed joy. We sang our songs, I rested a lot in the car or in people's guest rooms, and then we headed home.

The night we arrived home, we had a haphazard dinner—I call it "a little of this, little of that". Drives the boys crazy when I say that. And we listened to Connor tell us funny stories about his wrestling team and practices. He was trying wrestling for the first time, and loved the way it helped him get in shape, to be both strong and flexible. But as he said, "I don't have the 'heart' of a wrestler, Mom. I'm not into it enough to really be fierce at it." However, when I saw him at his first match, I had to put my coat over my head as I saw him grapple with his opponents head and neck and his long legs pushing them both around on the mat. Hmm. I guess I don't have the heart of a wrestler's mother.

Anyway, we had our dinner and we were happy and we were all going to bed, and I had one of those absolute "aha", light bulb moments while brushing my teeth. I remembered that, during the first round of illness, someone had written on the website that when she had been sick, she had wondered "why me?" but she also heard the same inner voice ask "why NOT me?" I suddenly thought of all the people on this planet thought, of course! Why NOT me? Of all the billions of people, why should I be exempt, if everybody is not exempt? It was like a piece of a puzzle falling into place, and some of my anxiety and despair fell away.

At about 10 A.M. the morning of February 6, I received a call from Jay, the Bone Marrow Transplant coordinator, who reported that everything was ready for me to be admitted the next day. He reminded me about where to go to register (as if I needed reminding) and a few other details. I spent the day e-mailing, calling my sisters, and packing. At about 3:00 that afternoon, Jay called back and said there may be a delay because my insurance company was refusing to pay for the transplant. They would not, more specifically, pay for the "mini". They would pay for the more conventional transplant, where I would undergo more serious chemotherapy, would have a greater chance of dying, and would require a longer hospital stay, but not for the non-myoablative procedure, because it was deemed too "experimental". Well, there is so much literature that even the average lay person can read volumes that speak to the contrary. This is not experimental anymore, and it is so much less harrowing on the patient, how could one NOT choose that option, if given the choice?

This was impossible. I was to go in the <u>next day</u> and they were just now telling us this? It was unconscionable. But when I thought about it, it seemed my case manager had been a little vague in the last one or two phone conversations; in fact, she had told me she would be out of town this week, so when I tried to call her, I was referred to another extension on which I could leave a message for the man taking her calls. "Hello answering machine, may I please speak to … my insurance company?" It's a giant company…who to talk to? I was almost hysterical. I wanted so much for the planned admission to take place because it felt so right. The arithmetic of it all fit: I would go in on the 7th, have the transplant on the 14th, and my real birthday is on the 21st. So it all was happening in multiples of seven, and the transplant on Valentine's Day?? Come on! That was just too perfect. So I spoke up a little louder than I usually do, and I was heard. Jay called back and relayed a message from Dr. Nelson who felt sure that this would be a short period of conflict and we should go ahead and admit me as planned; he would handle my insurance company. So we were back on track, and would begin the transplant prep the next day. I was going in.

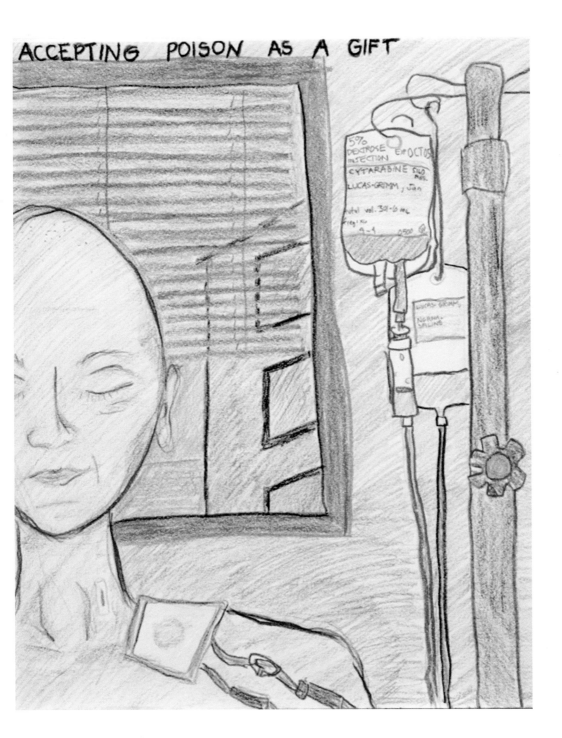

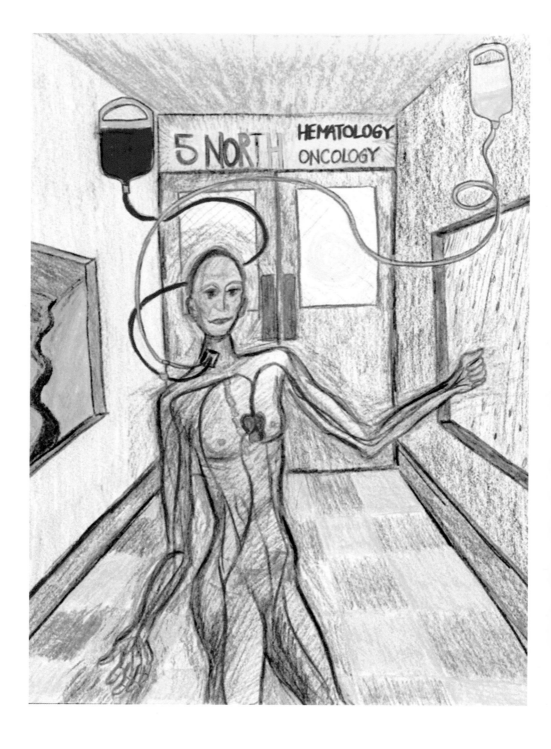

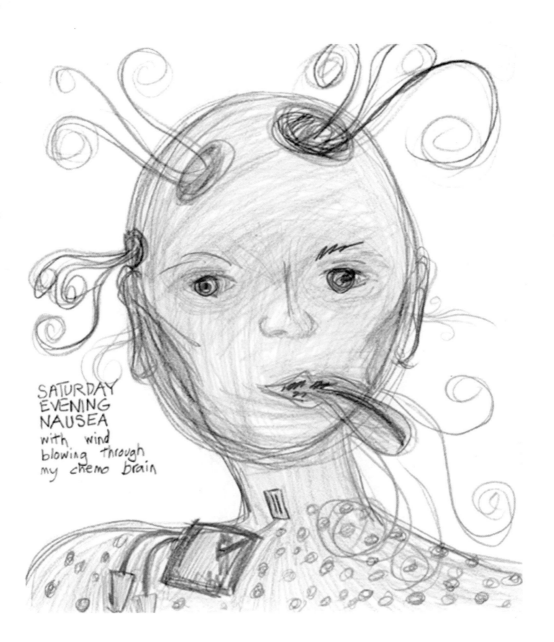

SATURDAY
EVENING
NAUSEA
with wind
blowing through
my chemo brain

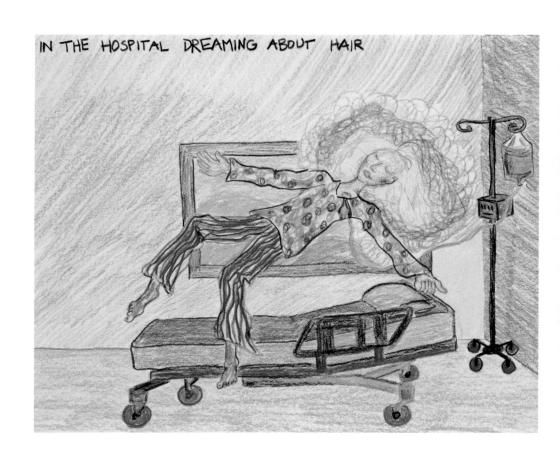

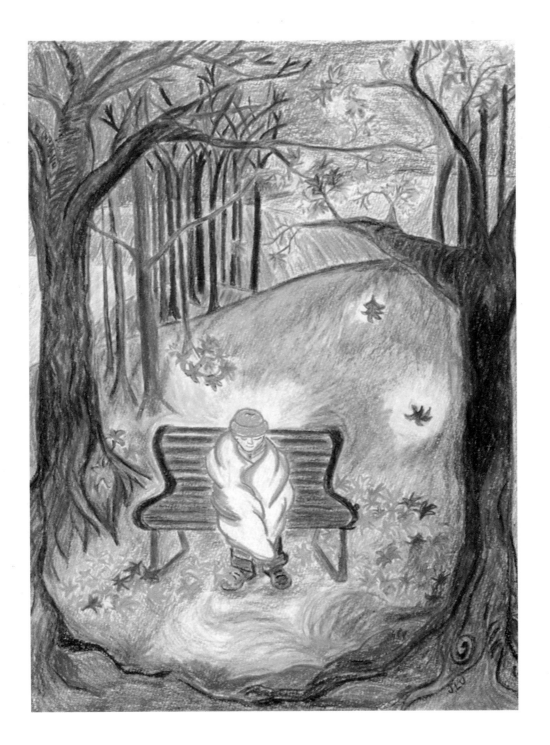

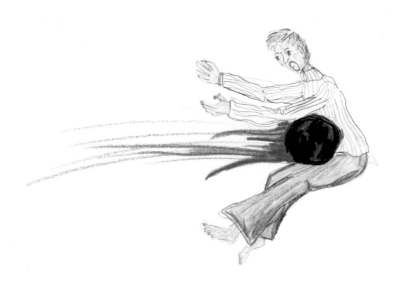
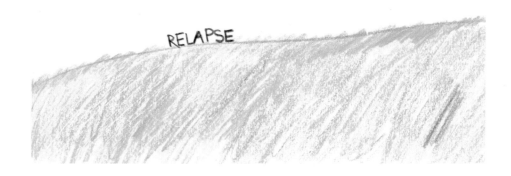

RELAPSE

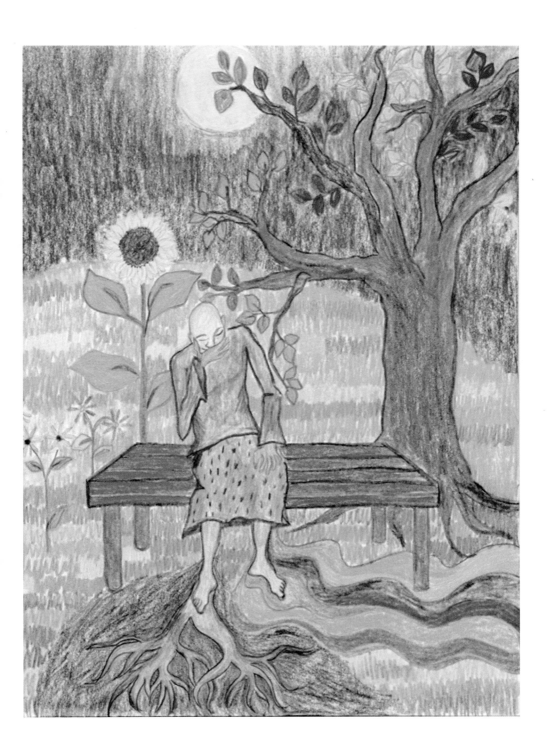

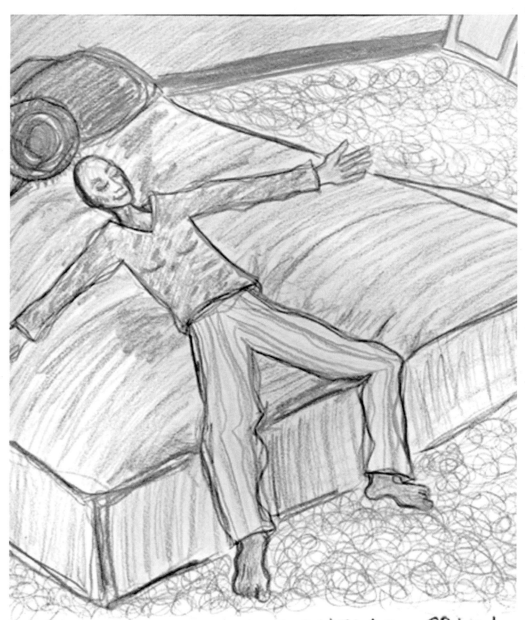

BLUE GIRL WITH CHEMO BRAIN
ON HER OWN BED

⊛ Inishfree

Ireland Music Tours

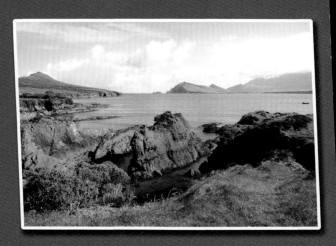

Tours for people who hate tours!

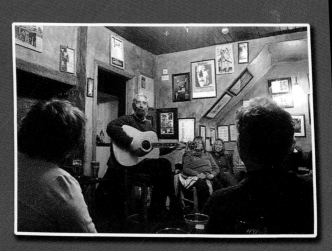

Relaxed ⊛ *Intimate* ⊛ *Flexible*

Welcome to In

Ireland moves at its own pace, and if you

How can you see a lot of Ireland but see it at Ireland's pa
without feeling like just another face in the big-tour cro
special tours.

Inishfree's tours are created for people who hate tours.
groups or hurried stops. What you will have is a wonder
and culture that Ireland has to offer.

By day we take in the incredible sights: castles, cottages
dolmens, rugged coastlines with crashing waves and ca
hedgerows and a thousand shades of green.

By night we wine and dine and take in the amazing sou
the 'craicin' sessions of classic pubs—where local players
bodhráns and uilleann pipes, and a tall tale or two.

With Inishfree Ireland Music Tours, you're not just anoth

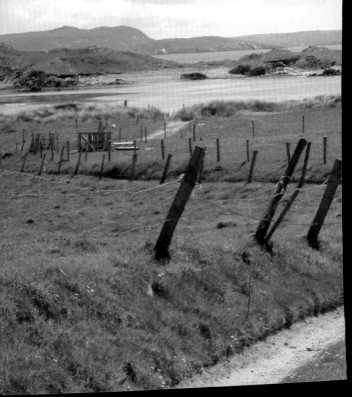

8

I *was welcomed the morning* of February 7th by Kelly, the nurse I had met previously when Dr. Bob had taken me on a tour of the transplant unit. She is so sunny and lovely it was positively contagious. She acted as if she had been looking forward to my arrival and I was finally there. It felt so different than the last time I had been in the hospital, when I had relapsed. That was not planned for and was very depressing. Again I was in to do a very hard thing, but this time I was very prepared. And I was so comforted by the nurses and all the surroundings. As I had noticed before, I was struck by how our environment affects us. The rooms in the BMT unit are newer and beautifully appointed; there is nice tile on the walls and in the big bathroom (with a <u>flush toilet</u> and a big shower!!), as well as a glass cabinet in which one can put mementos from home, and even the lighting was warm and welcoming. There are large, framed close-up photographs of flowers on the walls of the rooms and hallways. It felt so much more civilized and soothing then the old part of the hospital. I thought, "This will be home for a good long while, I guess. That's the plan."

I received a second round of chemo the next afternoon and then started on an immune suppressant in preparation for the new cells. I was talking to my bones, telling them to be a good home for the new cells. On average, it takes about 12 days for the Graft versus Host (GVH) to show up. GVH is the condition in which the donor cells react badly to the host tissue. It commonly affects the skin, the mouth, and even the digestive tract. I instructed my bones have very good manners and welcome the new guys, "Hi, how are you doing? Come on in, make yourselves comfortable, we are so glad to have you here, in fact we <u>love</u> you…"

Sometimes when you're in a hospital room, it is easy to think of all the life happening out there in the world without you. You think of everybody driving around and working and cooking and eating and drinking (Guinness, dammit) and sweeping and shopping…all the stuff of life. In the hospital, however, life is telescoped down to a few activities: eat breakfast, brush teeth, walk in the hallway, read a bit, get ready for lunch, brush teeth, walk in the hall… you see where this is going. It's a smaller universe and it is easy to feel alone. But when I read all the e-mail (and snail mail) and I knew people really were thinking about me, it made me feel a part of the larger world still and for that, I was so grateful.

By February 10, it was beginning to feel a lot like chemo…nausea and that general achy feeling that comes with the onslaught of chemicals. But so far, my trusty friend and drug of choice, Atavin, was doing the trick to keep the baddies at bay. I had a deluxe exercise bike in the room and the large bathroom felt spa-like. My docs were sort of biding their time before the Big Day; they stopped by to chat and we discussed their kids, my kids, some technical bladiblah that I sort of understood, and the weather. No politics. I was grateful for their company and their conversation.

This really was a waiting game. I didn't even feel like I needed to be in the hospital. I just had occasional nausea, and I knew how to deal with that. The doctor explained to us that should this "mini" become the norm, and there are divided schools of thought on the matter, this part of the prep could happen at home. That way I could be getting the medicine at home, preparing for the harder part ahead.

One of those days, walking back and forth in the hallway, I happened to notice that sunshine was flooding in on the other side of the floor, whereas my side of the hallway was darker and shadowy, especially in my corner room which faced out to the back of the parking lot. So I inquired about the one empty room on that side, and a few hours later, I was in it! What a difference. Not only was there more light, but the construction of the new cancer center was right outside my window and there were interesting things to watch all day. Quite entertaining, although I did agree with one of the nurses who wished it was summer and the workers would have had their shirts off.

I was knitting like a mad woman, although Atavin seemed to be creating new stitches, and I was muddling through crossword puzzles. The Olympics were the highlights of my TV viewing. I missed Tim and the boys on such a deep level it was hard to deal with. I just wanted to have a good dose of their smells; even the dog's who, by the way, always smells great. I was yearning to run my hands through those boys' blondish heads of hair, and give them big hugs when they were least expecting it. I had a deep craving for them. Tim got a little worried that I was only on Day Five of so many more days and I was already hankering for home. I think it was because I didn't really feel sick and it was my sixth hospitalization. It was easy to forget that I was in there for the really big deal, the transplant. I just wanted my family, and my kitchen, and my bedroom, filled with their voices and the general clatter of home.

It was truly a countdown and I felt the energy of my community of supporters carrying me along. On February 13, my sister Pat arrived and ensconced herself in the University Hotel to stay with me during the transplant and for two weeks after. I kept thinking, in the very back of my mind, that someone was going to come in and tell me that my donor had gotten sick or had decided not to go through with it, or something. I had been warned so many times that it was such a balancing act with so many factors to line up just so, that I could just imagine a piece of the puzzle not fitting. In fact, a large part of the BMT staff was going to Hawaii that very day for a conference about transplants. Thank heaven Dr. Bob was not planning on going, but many of the other doctors, as well as the transplant coordinator, were planning their trip and were to depart February 14.

Pat came to my room on the morning of The Day and we tried to act normal as the day progressed. We played a word game over and over and Pat tried to get me to get into Sudoku, but to no avail. I was a crossword nut and so pleased that I could still do them (barely) even in my post-chemo state. But nobody that I know personally can do a crossword faster than my sister Pat. She does the *New York Times* Sunday puzzle in ink, in about an hour or less, so she's my hero in that regard. Well, in many regards, but in crosswords for sure! So we carried on that day, knowing that Tim would be up later in the day and he was touching base with us hourly for any news.

I also knew that there was to be a gathering of friends at the Unitarian Church to send along love and prayers and meditations and good energy, healing energy, my way. They were going to have a bonfire and drink red wine and eat good food, which Unitarians are known for, and just have a real valentine lovefest! I felt sort of left out actually. I knew they were meeting at about 5:30. At that time, Pat had gone back to her hotel to change and freshen up, and Tim was home having dinner with the boys and I knew everyone was elsewhere with someone. So I moped around for a bit, feeling very alone, and then decided to go to the website and read the guestbook. I just sat there, in my pretty little room with all my decorations and pictures and I drank in every message on the website and I wept. I sat there and wept. All the amazing and lovely people thinking of me, wondering about my ordeal, wishing they could do something for me, and sending all that over the Internet! It was truly amazing. I wiped my eyes, smiled to myself, told myself to buck up and got back into bed to wait. Then Pat came back to the room, and said since all the people were gathering to send me good vibes, <u>we</u> should do something too. So, not being too new-agey or anything, we held hands and squeezed our eyes shut, and said "thank-you" to everything and everyone.

We realized that probably early that morning, my donor would have been in a hospital somewhere getting blood drawn out of her, the stems cells being spun out and separated, and the rest of her blood being returned into her via a different line. Those cells would be stored in a blood bag, just like a transfusion bag, put in a cooler, and transported here. They were scheduled to arrive at the hospital between 10 and 11 P.M. that night. They would go first to the lab for some kind of analysis and then they would come upstairs to BMT and get infused into me. That could be around 12 or 1 in the morning. All the nurses and docs said it was rather anti-climatic because it's just another bag hanging off my IV pole and nothing earth shattering happens right away. ("Anti-climatic for you maybe!!" I was thinking.)

The nurses said it's like getting a new birthday; now I will have two. February 14th takes on a whole new meaning. The cells will float around for a while when they first enter my vascular system. Then they will migrate to my bones and begin to differentiate into the cells they will become—the various kinds of blood making cells and immune cells, like neutrophils. When they get to my bones and decide to set up housekeeping, that's called "engrafting". This process takes up to two weeks, and we would know it was happening by my rising white counts. At that moment, my white count was almost down to zero. I asked why I didn't feel sick if my white count was so low and the doctor said it's because of the way we got there. Unlike past treatments, which included massive amounts of chemo to wipe out everything, this had been more gradual and because I had been in remission, they were not trying to kill leukemia cells, just prevent any new ones. So, all in all, this first leg of the journey was relatively easy.

Once while walking in the hall, I met a patient from Fargo, North Dakota and there were a few others from far away. I learned that this is one of THE places to come for a bone marrow transplant. How amazingly lucky that I live so close. The sun was pouring in my window as I watched the construction of the new cancer center down below. Lots of Olympics to watch and crossword puzzles to do while we waited. Tim finally arrived after having a really good dinner with the boys. He said they all discussed the procedure and that both boys were feeling very comfortable with all of it, very confident that I would be well. Then we got women's curling on the Olympics channel (am I the only person in Indiana who loves curling?) and every once in a while, one of us would say, "I wonder where the cells are now? Are they on a plane? Are they on the ground?" Tim began to nod off, Pat's head was dropping down occasionally, but I was wide awake. At one point we got a phone call from one of the transplant nurses saying, "The cells are in the building. They have to go to the lab, and then they'll be on their way to you." Well, that news woke everyone up. At 11:30 P.M. we heard from outside the door, a voice calling out, "Ta-Da!!" Two nurses and the stem cell lab woman entered and said "We're here!!!" And there they were: one woman was holding a little Igloo Cooler with a little flattish bag of pink creamy-looking liquid inside, the other two smiling excitedly as they entered. They went through the check-in, verifying numbers and my arm bracelet, and then they handed me the bag! My new life was right there in that little blob of liquid. Tim took my picture with my new cells and I kissed the bag. The best part was that everybody in the room was into the spirit of the thing. The nurses were excited, Tim was snapping photos and it was all very celebratory and momentous. They hooked up the bag to my port and we watched as the strawberry colored liquid slowly made it's way through the long tubing. As it came closer and closer to entering my chest, we grew more and more excited. When it was about an inch from "entry", Tim took a picture and as it finally rounded the last curve and slipped into my blood stream, we cried. Pat and I cried, the nurses cried, Tim took pictures and the nurse who was in charge said it never failed to amaze her when this moment happened—after all her years of doing this, it still amazed her. I sat for about three hours as the liquid inched its way in. I was about ten minutes from the end of the infusion when I began to itch. I looked at my arms and legs: <u>hives</u>. Oh-no... I remembered this—been there, done that, and did NOT want a repeat of the itch-fests of the old days. So I breathed very carefully, deeply and slowly, Pat pressed on my head and shoulders, and finally the last of it went in and they gave me anti-itch meds plus a muscle relaxant. I was out like a light.

The next morning was Day +1. We began the count from there. The first 100 days are the key marker of a certain level of success. From Day +1 on, I would be taking two immune suppressants and three antibiotics and my immune system would be quite vulnerable. I had to realize that it would be the time for masked visitors and books and movies. I would watch Spring emerge from a distance this time— no more running in the fields like last year.

Valentines Day would never be the same and I would never be the same (in fact, my blood type has changed and I will eventually have to be immunized all over again). As I look back on that day, the transplant day, I am almost in disbelief at the miracle of it all. Think of it: someone else's cells entering a new body and starting to do the work they are genetically programmed to do! It was kind of wonderful and kind of spooky to wake up the next morning and know this had taken place. It was almost like a dream because I didn't feel any different. Jack asked me that day on the phone if my skin looked pinker or if my face looked red. I told him that I had wondered the same thing that morning and had thrown off my blankets and looked at my legs and arms to see if I could see evidence that something had happened. I was looking for a sign, I suppose. The next couple of days, as I would walk out in the hallway, I would wonder if it actually "took". I really wondered if maybe it had just gone right through me or something, because I felt nothing different. I asked Dr. Nelson, who I was now calling Dr. Bob, if he was sure the transplant had "taken" and was working. He said he was sure. Now we would watch the "chimerism", which was the ratio of my old cells to the new cells. The idea was that the new cells would overtake the old ones and start reproducing themselves. This could be confirmed by blood tests and eventually by a bone marrow biopsy. My friends were as intrigued by the process as I was. Sue and Darryl sent me the poem "Miracles" by Walt Whitman, and the line: "to me every hour of the light and the dark is a miracle" rang like a bell in my heart. I was a walking miracle!

9

One morning Dr. Bob walked in and sat down in one of my armchairs to talk with my sister and me. We were chatting about a variety of things and I just sort of waited for him to talk about my "status". He got around to it without segue, as is his want, and told me that my new cells were entering the lymph system right about then and that I needed to welcome them. He told me that the cells need to feel welcome, but that they need to know that I am in charge and that they cannot behave like unruly children. He said that they are going to want to say, "Where the heck are we? What are we doing here?" He said I would need to let them know that they are here to stay and to just make themselves comfortable and get ready to work. "Use that imagery when you are talking to your cells." (How did he know I was talking to my cells?) I loved it that such a brilliant medical mind as his could actually perceive that I needed a metaphoric way to understand the process, and that he spoke my language.

One other day, he had been trying to explain T-cell differentiation to Pat and me, and although he endeavored to use lay terms, his understanding was so complex that when he left we just looked at each other and shook our heads in bewilderment. We tried to remember what he had just said, but our recall could not handle all that information. He was just too smart for us! I wrote in the journal:

> So that's the guy who is in charge of my recovery, along with all the other members of the team. I am so lucky. I have to do my part, which involves drinking lots of fluids, eating as best I can, walking the halls and riding the exercise bike. Yesterday I was jogging in the halls and caught a glimpse of myself in a win-

dow and I remembered how self-conscious I was when I was first admitted. Now I parade around in a duckbill mask without flinching and I forget that I am bald… how priorities change over time. I am certain that all our combined energies that went towards welcoming my cells on 2/14 helped everything to go smoothly. Keep those cells in your thoughts and prayers so they don't misbehave. I will do my best to remain in charge. -Jan

It was a pretty easy going time, another waiting game in a way: waiting to see/feel GVH, wondering if the littlest ache or itchy feeling was the beginning of something bigger. I was of two minds about this: if I had no GVH, I would certainly feel better, and also be less worried that it would seriously affect my organs. On the other side of the issue, a little GVH indicates that the new cells are active and doing "their thing".

The worst thing that happened was that my "plumbing" slowed down, way down. I hadn't been consuming enough water in general, and my stomach was sticking out like a hard melon and getting bigger! Finally, after a couple of different suggestions, the nurse brought me a sucrose-type drink. It was better than the fizzy stuff I had tried to get down earlier, to no avail, but it was a thick, viscous liquid and difficult to swallow. The down side, they told me, was that I might have some cramping. SOME? Yikes. It did the trick, but it was painful getting there, like small herds of elephants were walking around inside me. I learned my lesson, and kept a full tumbler of water on hand at all times. I drank a little bit all day long and that solved the problem.

The doctors were watching my blood counts every day, to see if the cells were taking hold. It reminded me of the first time I had been waiting for neutrophils. I had assumed that my cells would recover in record time, and I felt the same way about the new cells. I assumed they would be charging ahead and I would go down in the medical history books for the fastest post-transplant cell takeover EVER. Once again, I had to get back to reality.

I would walk the hallways, back and forth, and back and forth, with my sister Pat. We would try not to stare, but we could tell that many of the rooms held very seriously ill patients, and we would look at each other or squeeze each other's hands, just a quiet thank-you for my relatively good state of health. Pat would bring me an occasional frozen dinner entrée but I was craving different foods, most particularly, fresh carrots. I even asked the nutritionist to come up and talk to me about this. I was pretty sure I could sway her mind, but No, she was adamant that I eat from the neutropenic kitchen and my vegetables must be cooked. Cooked to within an inch of mush, mind you. I imagined various dinners I would have when I got out: fresh green salads with exotic cheeses, like Roquefort and Gorgonzola, sourdough breads, grilled steak and pork chops, and maybe some more vegetables for dessert. My cravings were starting to become obsessive! I dreamed about food, I wrote about food and I drew pictures of food.

Pat reported in from the outside world, which was miserably cold and icy. She did my laundry, brought me candy bars (not exactly on the menu but okay since they were packaged), and played a zillion games of Upwards with me. This is a game like Scrabble in 3-D and you can put tiles on top of others to make new words. We were pretty obsessed with it, and I still have the sheets of paper we used to score. I like the proof that, even though she is the crossword champ of the family, I could actually beat her at a word game. We were both amazed that my chemo-addled brain could call up any words and beat her. But let the records show: I was the winner overall. Thank God, because my brain was, and still is, a bit foggy.

I was having another birthday in the hospital, uggh. Apparently I had a knack for hitting the holidays. The celebration was low-key, since I had already celebrated the "cell" birthday. Tim brought the boys up and they presented me with a new pair of shoes, ones that were a light blue version of the very shoes they had bought for themselves! I was honored to be in that company in terms of style. Lucas came down from Chicago and actually spent the night at the hospital. No "Blue Chair" though. He had to have a cot set up in the lobby/waiting room of the clinic and he slept there. The next day he came into my room early, blurry-eyed, and fell asleep promptly on my bed, as I sat in the chair and read. It was great just to have him there and watch him sleep.

I am known in some circles for my love of birthdays (especially my own). I have never been shy about celebrating, throwing myself parties, and making it widely known when the day arrives. So the people who knew that about me, and even those who didn't, were turning up the volume on the website.

One of my friends wrote me that she had noticed my willingness to be healed. "Willingness to be healed..." what an interesting way to think about it. But it's true, this healing game is not a passive exercise and it is not something you can be dragged into either. You must be willing, and I think, actively involved. I am still, as of this writing, actively involved in my healing and occasionally need to be reminded of that fact. It seems like this is the way it will be for the rest of my life. I wish I could convey this to my children, but they don't see themselves as anything but strong, healthy, immortal. The specter of illness or death eludes them, even though they have been walking this journey with me. They are young and completely focused on the now, the way they look, the way they walk, the way they perceive others to be looking at them. It's kind of beautiful because they are teenagers and that's what teenagers are supposed to do. But I can only hope that this experience has informed them, deep inside, of the absolute necessity of taking good care of their health.

"Without health, all riches mean nothing." Some wise person said that, or something like it, a long time ago. I remember reading it as a young person and thinking, no, riches could go a long way even if you weren't healthy. But later I realized, no—<u>being</u> healthy enables you to enjoy things—riches or family or a beautiful day. Now, especially, I know how health and the feeling of well being informs my every thought, my every action. And we are all in various states of <u>healing</u>, I think, the older we get. Our bodies have weathered sickness, injury, childbirth, stress, whatever we have been through takes a toll, and so healing is an ongoing process. It seems so obvious when you're sick, that you need to heal. But when we're well and dashing around hell-bent for leather that we forget that we need to heal, take care, be well.

So, as we monitored the cells, the chimerism, it was ascertained that my donor cells were at 30% while my old cells were hanging in there at 70%. I wanted the ratio to be different, of course, but the verdict arrived suddenly: I could go home. Yikes! Once again, I could hardly wait to be back in my living room and at the same time, I was nervous about leaving my team of nurses and doctors. Another departure, another step, another ride home.

TUESDAY, FEBRUARY 28—I am writing from the sunny sunroom (aptly named) in our HOME!!! I AM HOME. Let me back up: on Saturday, I had some weird and painful stomach aches and the doctor wasn't sure if it was gastritis or GVHD, the graph versus host disease that could rear it's head at any moment. He checked in on me about five times, gave me the special stomach coating liquid that made me barf (not the desired effect), then we went to mundane over-the-counter antacid, and it did the trick. My white counts continued to steadily climb, the pains were under control, and Sunday afternoon, Dr. Bob said, "I think you can go home tomorrow." My sister Pat and I promptly freaked out. First elation, then terror, then the feeling that I had to get out that instant, then back to being nervous about leaving that safe little cocoon. It was the thought of fresh carrots that kept me moving forward. As I was wheeled down to the front door of the hospital while Tim went to get the car, I had this complete déjà vu feeling…I've left that hospital SIX times now, and I prayed inwardly that it would be my last. But the reality is that there is an 80% chance that I will have to be readmitted for something, be it a small fever or cough or whatever. Then, as we left the circle drive and headed home, I cried. I couldn't stop! It's just so intense, going in and out of that place. I am so lucky and so grateful and so sick of being sick. I just wonder at my stamina…will I be able to keep on keeping on? At least a good cry seems to alleviate my nausea so I feel it is not only okay but actually good and helpful for me to have a big weep now and again.

So, home. Once again I'm amazed by things. Like trees. On the drive home, through the grayish green landscape of the dormant fields, you can see the trees so well and there are so many. I mean, they just keep growing, they come right up out of the ground and grow for so long, regardless of wars or leukemia or the presidents who come and go or households that occupy the land for a while, and then new ones arrive. And our house is beautiful and healing and I ate a salad with many carrots and sugar snap peas and I plan to lay on the couch for the rest of the day, with my phone and antacid nearby. The beginning of a new phase.

The BMT booklet reads, "You have not reached the top of a mountain, only a plateau. The view may be lovely but the terrain is still bumpy and you have a ways to go." So, I see Dr. Bob on Friday. I have a port still hanging out of my lower neck and I have to flush it out with saline everyday and Tim has to change the dressing twice a week. Whoever thought we'd become so facile with the medical stuff…and me with the lingo! Yikes, I could pass for a doctor.

But I don't think I will. I am drawing and writing and resting and I'm back on the Leukemia Couch, as we call it. It will have to be burned in a ritual pyre of healing and wellness someday. But that's down the road. One step at a time. Thank you for everything, all of you. -Jan

10

The *website began a saga* that certainly took all our minds off cancer. It was decided, since I was spending so much time on my couch, that all the friends out there in the wide world of the web should too. That way, they could send all that energy they weren't using cleaning houses or doing whatever productive thing they were supposed to do, to me! Thus began the "Couch Tales", apparently spurred on by the memory of some other historical couch sitters known as the Baumgartners. So not only were the websiters talking to each other, an entire sub-culture was arising! The caringbridge site had given way to a cult of couch worshippers—or couch-burners? I couldn't always exactly figure out where the metaphor was going. I knew it had something to do with giving me extra energy, through saving their own? Were they sitting on their couches that are already on the porch? Or going to take them put there, in preparation for the ritual burning? It was a bit confusing but very funny and I was happy to be on the edges of the attention. I wanted everybody there, not talking just about me. Talking about me usually meant I was sick, and so I loved the freedom from that and what it meant. It was so funny to read about. It was as if a wave of creativity had been loosed from these long-time friends and in some ways, we were all our best selves, again.

There was still nausea, and port maintenance, and the weekly clinic visit. There were long days on the couch with naps and phone calls and walks with the dog. There were also new aches in my joints and muscles that positively scared me. I remembered this feeling…it was the feeling I had had in January and February of 2005. It was like a shadow of the old illness was living inside of me and I couldn't shake it. Dr. Bob put me on prednisone for the pain and it miraculously disappeared. But that feeling of knowing…of recognizing the deep bone pain and thinking about what it could be was exceptionally unnerving. It turned out, and has over the years, that many of those old pains reoccur but they don't mean the same thing. In other words, the bone pain that I remember feeling before initial diagnosis is a very similar pain that presented itself as GVH. Different reasons, same pain. Scary.

One of the frequent contributors to the website was my friend Maribeth. She was an avid couch-sitter, but more importantly, she was often my barometer of how "things were going" and how they were going to be. She had been at her teenage son's side for almost two years after doctors discovered a rare tumor in his leg and they had been in and out of University of Chicago Children's Cancer Center for some time. She was the consummate champion for her son's treatment, never ceasing in her questions and vigilance and I was often quite cheered by their news. He had undergone a stem cell transplant and at 16, was struggling with very different issues, such as school and friends and teen-age things. But he was still a fellow human with this weird disease, as was I, and I followed his progress with interest. He had a website also, and I wrote him a few times. I also heard through his aunt, my dear friend and artistic colleague, about his progress. They were well-versed in the cancer lingo and knew the ropes.

So, couches or no couches, my recovery was proceeding along, mostly in a rather bumpy fashion. Some days I was curled on the couch fighting nausea, other days I could take walks and draw, and feel a bit of energy growing on the inside. I went to see Dr. Bob, and one of the many reasons I was so fond of him was that he listened to every single symptom and description of every single feeling I had. I underwent a major check-up: blood work, which was all fabulous, and then had a bone marrow biopsy, the results of which would come in about five days. Dr. Bob said my case was rather unusual because he'd never seen anyone's platelets return to normal so fast; that, and all my numbers were right on track, just faster. He seemed so pleased and I, of course, started to worry: maybe it didn't "take", maybe I had too many platelets from the old cells, were the new ones working yet???

After that appointment, my friend Mary had to wheel me out to the car in a wheelchair because I was still loopy from the sedative. Which was all well and good until we got halfway home and realized I hadn't filled my prescription and it could only be filled at the hospital. So back we went, and as Mary was running up to get the pills, I stayed in the car. Well, of course, someone needed to get their car out and we were in the way, so I had to move Mary's car. I slid over to the drivers seat and looked for the gear shift. Where was it? I was turning on the wipers and blinkers and the washer spray and looking over at the waiting driver who was peering in at me. I waved and smiled, my bald head glinting in the sun. "Hi hi, no problem, just a sec!" Just then Mary raced out and took over the wheel and we left the place once again. Then without much warning, well, enough to open the car door, I started barfing. Lots. We turned the corner and there were all the construction guys working on the new Cancer Center, and I stuck my bald head out and heaved for a good long while. I wanted to tell them, "See? You're building this new place for people like me!" I think it was the morphine. That, and the non-stop snacking of the morning on pea pods, cheese and crackers and carrots! Lots of carrots.

I was so happy to be eating fresh veggies again. So happy to see my dog, who had been quite disgruntled with me. So happy to curl up on the Leukemia Couch and rest and draw and read trashy women's magazines (who in God's name can wear those clothes, much less afford them??) Liz had been by, helping me with everything, Dave and Cathy were doing laundry for me, Janeo was cooking, Carol knit me an orange hat...just the color I craved those Spring days, everybody was driving my boys all over the place and everyone on the website was so funny! I loved everybody...and the thing is: I really did. I had reason to. Love was in the air; love and life and healing.

Spring was definitely coming. You could hear the peepers at night, those tree frogs that sound like birds. Birds were really starting to make noise and my poor dog looked at me woefully to take him on a walk. But getting walked by him was too much. I could walk twice around the house with my attractive "duckbill" mask on or down the lane and back, then back to the Couch. I must say I was having a teeny bit of deja vu because this time the previous year I was coming home and so hopeful and so sure that the leukemia was just a little blip on the big screen of my life. Well, it ended up being quite a bit more than that and the relapse was so hard to accept. I just tried meditating on my sweet cells, to keep them working and happy with no thoughts of defection. But I did wonder sometimes—what if??— I couldn't help it. That's when I would turn to the website or to friends or even just to my own memories and crack up or smile or cry and forget my worries, and just kiss the moments as they came. I wrote:

> Hey couch women... I'm sure the solidarity with my cells re- clining helps me heal. Although I'M reclining; they're work- ing hard. I saw Dr. Nelson yesterday and he says numbers are great and that my bone marrow (from the biopsy) is "BEAU- TIFUL". He said there are no blasts and it's healthy, red and juicy. He also said that of 55 "mini" transplants they have done at IU there have been no relapses. My usually upbeat mind took a small journey to the Dark Side because I remember such upbeat conversations over on 5-N last year: "you're the wellest sick woman we've ever seen" and "you're going to beat this, no problem". And then what happened? RELAPSE. Aaaah, remisssion...it's an iffy word. I would have to say that my re- lapse last fall was more difficult than the first diagnosis and the possibility of it happening again lurks around in the corners of my day sometimes. I told Dr. Nelson about this and he said it's perfectly normal but perfectly useless; to please try and get hold of the negative feelings and sweep them away and focus on the moment, on my cells doing their lovely work, and on health. He recommends shiatsu...I love that. So it's up and down out here on the farm. It's rainy and cold, which prevents me from walking outside. I am a complete weeny; the littlest breeze chills me through and through like I'm a sieve. I walk around the house and try to stretch and then the couch or the bed call to me...so I respond. It's a bumpy road. xxxooo -J

11

It was an interesting time. "Interesting" is often a word we use when we don't want to say how really bad or difficult a thing is, like saying to an actor after her performance: "Hmmm, well, the play was…interesting." Dealing with leukemia and chemo, and then the specific act of transplant, was clear-cut. Now the variations in what could possibly happen post-transplant were harder to understand. And my usual attitude of "well, it won't happen to me—I'll be the one exception to the rule" wasn't necessarily going to work. Things were in a gray area. I continued to report in on the website:

> Rain, this Indiana rain. It's kinda driving me loony. It's really a pretty dismal aspect of winter here and it is definitely hampering my walking. I finally bundled up with coats, scarf, two hats, socks, pants, boots, gloves and the ever-lovely duck-bill mask to top it off. I sloshed partway down the lane and even that little bit made me feel good. A person's gotta move her legs! I'm compiling my list of healing helps: walking (everyday, at least once a day, even if you REALLY don't want to), fresh veggies, good music, laughter (any way you can get it, and that includes 13-year-olds' scatological jokes), scribble or draw or cut paper and glue…get back to some elementary kind of art activity that you knew you were good at…back then. (You are still good at it but you don't know that.) Eat some treats now and again but drink lots of water so you don't any plumbing problems…oh listen to me! OY—enough with the aches and pains and laxatives talk. On other notes, I am figuring out how

to navigate the headache and to draw some mean pictures if I feel down. Breathing seems to help the aches and the mean drawings will go in a drawer somewhere for another day. They're quite scary...tee-hee, -Jan

   I had a rather sobering visit with Dr. Bob. It seemed that the donor cells were only at about 30% in by bloodstream and my own cells are at 70%. So we needed to lift off some of the immune suppression to let the donor cells shake it up a bit more and do their thing. My first reaction was "I knew this was too good to be true! I knew I was feeling too well." One is always grateful to be feeling good but I knew that a certain amount of feeling bad was required to let us know that the cells were doing their thing. I had been preparing for the worst ever since I entered the hospital and the worst never came. I like having a job, however difficult, spelled out to me and then I'll DO IT but this waiting around to see if something's happening was very hard for me. Doctor Bob said it's a dance of balancing meds and cell activity, watching for pain indicators and other symptoms and dulling pain, etc. I would have liked a big flashing sign that said "everything's going well...cells are flourishing...they're slower than some but faster than others" and morning bulletins saying: "we had a good night, we're working hard, you can eat Roquefort cheese in two weeks"...stuff like that. I just wanted to KNOW what's going on. But alas, I couldn't. So I had to give over to the greater universe and trust that everything was unfolding as it should. Hah! I could do that about 1 minute a day...I had lost some of my Zen approach and I was just pissed that I actually had leukemia and I seemed to be crying a lot. But the couch phenomenon had me cracking up and I had to concentrate on renting funny movies and laughing, because what the hell else could I do?! I couldn't walk out in the cold wind and the rain and I had walked around and around our lovely house but I needed a change in the air. I decided I needed "I Love Lucy".

ST. PATRICK'S DAY—Kelly, one of the nurse practitioners for post-transplant patients, called with good news: it seems the donor cells have increased in the bloodstream to 76% and my old cells are going the way of the dinosaur!! She was very cute and excited when she told me. In order to avoid a massive case of Host vs. Graft, given the vigor of the cells right now, they increased the immune suppressant up to 100 mg 2x/day, half of where I started and twice what I took three days ago...so it is quite a balancing act and they will continue to monitor my blood and adjust meds up and down accordingly. Quite a relief. The cells must be working hard because I am exhausted! I am napping two times a day, often, and I'm beset by nausea which is a big pain. Nothing appeals, so it's back to liquid nutrition for a while and toast. Oddly enough, I can still eat baby carrots and sugar snap peas. Now I'm off to watch a DVD...I forget what it is...it doesn't matter...it's easy on the body. I am wearing my green Guinness shirt in honor of the day...I'll drink a bit extra when I'm well. You Chicagoans: have a drink for my cells, eh? And don't get near that green river!

I slept twice for an hour each yesterday and today for 2 1/2 hours after I'd been up just two hours! So much sleeping, and then it's hard to get up and then I started to feel just a wee bit sorry for myself, what to do? how long will this go on? will I ever ride my bike again? will I ever work again? will I ever whaaa whaaa whaaa. I tried the "mindfulness" exercises that the oncology therapist taught me and they gave me a headache. So I thought I'd get some real clothes on and go for a walk, but first I would take a look at the website. You guys make my heart sing, make me laugh out loud and cry from happiness and gratitude and freaking good fortune to have such support. You pick me up when I am falling. I have nothing to whine about now and will go out and walk, slowly, and breathe, and breathe, and help those beautiful cells along. -Jan

Hey no journal entry for a while because I've been barfing!!! whooopeee! The nausea developed into the real thing and finally, on Tuesday, I went to have my stomach and upper small intestine looked at, photographed and biopsied. We should get definitive results tomorrow or Monday. There doesn't seem to be evidence of GVHD though, but there IS evidence of some kind of "injury" that the stomach is recovering from...such as a virus. We'll know more later. I had the chance to talk to another bone marrow transplant guy...two years out from his transplant, and his words of advice were: take it easy, take it slow; this is like nothing you've ever done before and all your preconceived ideas of your big, strong, tough self have no meaning here (how did he know I felt that way?) He said your body is undergoing Transformation and that takes TIME, lots of it. So, couches, here I come. I am walking out in these beautiful warm days and I am drawing and even writing a tiny bit, and of course, there's another season of "West Wing" to soothe my furrowed brow. And even though it goes against my nature, I'm trying to sleep a lot and meditate and relax and just BE, not DO. -Jan

MARCH 30, 2006—Saw Dr. Nelson yesterday and it was uneventful...he says everything is moving in the right direction...slowly. My donor cells are up to 93% and he reduced the dose of one of the immune suppressors so that might stir up a bit of cell activity. Everything just seems so slow. It's beautiful outside and I'd like to be running with the dog and digging in the garden and messing around out there, but alas, not yet. I realize that I have to be moving at the Speed of the Body—like when you see microscopic footage on TV of blood moving or cells and they just are so tiny but they keep moving in these tiny little increments...that must be what's happening inside me. The cells are doing their thing at the speed of the body, not the speed of human life on the outside, which is frantic by comparison. So, I am s l o w i n g down. Still slightly woozy in the stomach and no appetite, which is absolutely depressing for a girl who likes to eat as much as I like to. But this too will pass. As you might imagine, the price of this whole ordeal is outrageous. Even though I'm lucky enough to have insurance, not everything is covered; there is a high deductible and high monthly premiums. The prescriptions alone are astronomical and the insurance covers a small portion of that. So my dear friends here have organized a most extraordinary benefit for our medical account: Carrie Newcomer and Jennie Devoe are doing a concert at the beautiful Indiana Repertory Theatre on April 30 at 7:00 P.M. These are two extraordinary singer-songwriters and they will be joined by my husband Tim Grimm as well. Also, my artwork (the Leukemia Art, as we call it) will be on display and for sale as well. Just what you want to cheer up your walls.

Well, actually, some of the pictures are quite hopeful, but as you might expect, some are kind of dark. But that's the experience and since I can't be there (can't be in crowded public places yet) I thought the art should be there to explain things. -Jan

Because of the upcoming benefit concert, our local newspaper wanted to do an article on me. The writer wanted to know some of my history, how I had fared from diagnosis up to the present, and the details of a bone marrow transplant. I was glad to be interviewed because I hoped to spread information about transplants. I thought it would be an ideal opportunity to explain how the transplant works and possibly encourage people to sign up to be donors. A photographer friend of ours took pictures for the article and I was confident it would be tasteful. I didn't know in advance when the article would come out so I hadn't said anything specific to Connor or Jack about it. Because our paper is delivered at the end of our long lane, we had not retrieved it before the boys had left for school the morning the article came out. Imagine their surprise when they got to school and most of the other kids had seen my picture, in full color and rather large, on the <u>front</u> page of the paper. The students were calling out, "Hey, you're famous!" or "Wow, I didn't know your mom had leukemia!" and other equally helpful comments. The boys were mortified. Of course, I didn't know any of this until they came home from school and I was sitting at the dining room table with the paper folded up next to me. They were both sort of sullen, but it was Jack who blurted out, "Why did you put your picture on the <u>front page</u>?" I was flabbergasted. "I didn't put it there, the newspaper people did. The editors decide what goes where, not me!" He didn't quite believe me. He thought it was like an advertisement we were making and that Tim and I chose to put my picture, in a bright orange fuzzy hat which covered up my bald head, on the front page. Then I asked him what was so embarrassing about the article. He said he didn't want us to be famous for having cancer. Bingo! Of course! I had to agree. I said, "Me neither! Jack, I'd rather be on the front page for having won a Tony award or for writing a prize-winning play. But the reality is that I did have leukemia and I did have a transplant, and if this can enlighten people about all that, then it's a good thing. Nothing to be embarrassed about." But the mind of an adolescent doesn't see things the way adults do, and they were both pretty ticked off about the whole thing. Just another way this was impacting their lives in ways I could not have imagined, and a reminder to keep checking in with them, because the depth of their feelings was far from obvious.

APRIL 18, 2006—Today was my weekly appointment with Doctor Nelson and he was reluctant to tell me that my donor cells have dropped down to 83%, so he has cut back one of the immune suppressants even more. We'll see if that helps things along. It kind of depressed me. I'm on Day +64 (post transplant) and I, of course, feel like it's been at least a year and REALLY wish I was further along in this process. Impatience will not help anything here though. It is a daily lesson and today it feels like I'm hitting my head against a wall. Spring is THE season to be in Indiana...it is so extravagantly beautiful right now. Little tiny green leaves on the trees cast a pale green veil over the woods and flowers on the redbuds and dogwoods, which are scattered all around our woods. There are no bugs yet and it's sunny and cool. I am really happy to be out in it and it saves my sanity to walk in the woods. I'm reading a lot and watching movies, such luxurious pastimes. That's the scoop from the BMT out in the country. I think I'm going to go have a talk with my cells... -Jan

APRIL 25—So the past four days have been fantastic—no stomach aches, lots more energy (not a single nap) and the weather was so beautiful that it was great to be out in it. Of course, as is my want, I unconsciously start to act as if everything's "normal"—I mean, I'm not running around like in the days of yore, but I DID start to feel like I was okay and I could, you know, drive around and drop the boys at their different places and walk the dog a LOT and my appetite is returning for a few things (jelly beans among others) and so I'm thinking: this must be good, very good. BUT as Dr. Nelson reminded me, this is a crucial time to hang tight, not overdo it, and that the patients who rush it at this point are the ones we LOSE!!! He actually SAID THAT! I said, "Lose??? Like...LOSE?" He nodded. Okay okay, I get the message. So while parts of my immune system are working, other parts are not and that it is so important to stay as well as possible. No infections or pneumonia for me—could be deadly. Then he said, "On another note, everything looks GREAT!" So-o-o-o, that was a cheery note, sort of like he was saying you're very close to the edge of the cliff, but you look really good there. Just another reminder that this is a very big transition for the body and just because I feel good, doesn't mean I am out of the woods. So it goes...life in the BMT lane. This, by the way, is the most amazing Spring I can remember here (not that I can remember anything) and I hope you all are getting to walk in a woods somewhere before it gets too leafy and humid or buggy and look at all the stuff coming out of the ground and out of the branches; it's truly amazing. It's an ecstatic moment before the onslaught of vegetation and we can really SEE everything right now. See it before it disappears into the woods! love, Jan

The benefit at IRT was an amazing event from all accounts; I guess I missed quite a party! Actually, I kind of felt like I was there because I received so many phone calls during the night from people who were there. "The audience is going in now...it's a lot of people." "Tim was great, so was James." "Jennie is amazing; I love her!" "Carrie Newcomer is awesome, her set was beautiful. I gotta go...they're all singing together!" I was getting a play by play as the night went on...it was really lovely to know that there was such a show of support and love of music and creativity and community. I hoped the message was heard about how easy it is to be a donor of stem cells. I wanted to spread the word about donating—it's all there on the National Bone Marrow Registry website. It's not painful, like it used to be, and it only takes a blood test to register.

> Okay, TODAY: saw Dr. Nelson. Today is Day +81 and my donor cells are back up to 93%. My lymphocytes are quite high so the immune suppressant has to go up too...we're adjusting the medicine weekly to achieve the balance that Dr. Nelson wants. But he went over some of the numbers with me (there are about 100 numbers he examines) and showed me how the trend has been going since March, which is basically great and he is very pleased. So, I left there feeling good and knowing that I HAVE to keep resting and just continue to enjoy the Spring. I am still ravenous a lot of the time, appetite is definitely coming back, yea!!! And walking with Satchel the Dog is good for me too. He walks me, actually. Patience has never been one of my virtues, but I am learning everyday. So, that's the news from BMT Olgilville, Indiana. Love, Jan

I still encounter people who were at the benefit, people I don't even know, and they tell me what a love-fest it was. It is still amazing to think about the effort and talent that went into making the evening not only successful in terms of our medical account, but a success in creating an entire evening of love and community and kindness. As I have been writing about this leukemia experience, from diagnosis and onward, that word keeps coming up: community. It is overused, no doubt, like *diversity*, or *globalization*, but it is undeniable: "community" arose around this illness, it arose to bring succor to those in need, and it turned out that those in need were...all of us! Not just the patient or the patient's family or the patient's friends. It turned out that we all needed each other, and we still do, and sometimes it takes things like a life-threatening disaster to bring us together. This illness made us all wake up for a time and see how much we care for each other, how much we need each other, and that it is all <u>worth it</u>. Only time will tell how long that stays with us. Memory fades with time, the intensity abates and everyday life rolls on. Hopefully, our detour off of the predictable path will stay with us in ways we can't foresee, a change that happened in our bones or our blood perhaps.

The weather was fabulous that Spring, with cool nights and mornings so the flowers on the dogwoods and locust trees were lasting a long time. My fingers were absolutely itching to get in the dirt and dig and pull weeds and plant. The garden was calling. So one Sunday, about fifteen other gardeners-friends-family heard the call and descended upon the land here and went to work, weeding, tilling, and putting in plants. It was extraordinary! I had to stay inside or wear my mask outside so the little molds and spores that are in the soil didn't find their way to my lungs. It was frustrating not to be digging too—usually my fingernails are dirty from May to October, but the gardeners results were lovely to behold. Many pots filled with beauteous annuals and the beds filled with perennials and borders of marigolds around everything. After everyone left, I just walked around and around the house and looked at it all. I sat on the porch and looked, and sat in the hammock and looked, and sat in the porch swing and looked and it was all a feast for the eyes. I was a lucky girl: to have this land where I could heal, to have friends and a community helping me along, and to be able to do things I loved while I was waiting for the body to do it's work. My skin felt like sandpaper and my eyesight seemed to be going downhill, but that was minor compared to all the life going on around and inside of me.

MAY 11, 2006—Did you ever think about your cells before? I sure didn't. But I am now and we all are a bit more aware, I bet. All that stuff going on in our bodies every second of every day, never stops working while we live, all the elements working together. Saw Dr. Nelson on Tuesday; Julie was my driver and appointment companion. She was as impressed as everyone always is with the fabulous doc and the nurses. My donor cells are 93%, the same for two weeks now, and Dr. Bob had expected a jump to 100% by now. So we're adjusting the meds again: off one of the immune suppressors altogether, and down to 75 mg. 2x/day from 100 mg. Right away, my skin started to itch and my bones and muscles ACHE! My body will adjust though, and then we'll see how it is next week. Dr. Bob said I could probably skip next week's appt if I was getting sick of coming up there and just get blood work done here in town. NOOO, I said. I need to come up and see him and be reassured. Truth is, I'm a little bit scared everyday and he is a bright spot in my week. The 21st of May is my 100th day and the Tuesday after that, I'll get a bone marrow biopsy and four hours of gamma globulin, so it'll be a big party all day up there. Whooopeee. Then, depending on results, I may skip a weekly visit...we'll see. I am nervous to skip a weekly visit; I'm kind of addicted to Dr. Bob.

We are going down to New Harmony for Memorial Day weekend and we're singing on the 27th in town...my first outing to sing since last November. I hope I remember how. Then, happily, Tim has a bunch of gigs all around Indiana for June and July so I'll sing with him when I can. That's the scoop from BMT Ogilville. Love, Jan

I started feeling really good, still napping, and eating everything in sight. Olives were like a drug—I couldn't stop eating them once I started. It reminded me very much of my pregnancies, when anything salty or vinegary tasted delicious. Summer vacation was right around the bend. My hammock would take the place of the couch, if I could keep Connor and Jack out of it. The flowers that the Garden Brigade had put in were doing beautifully and I was soaking up the healing energy they provided. I was planning on a slow, healing summer.

My donor cells seemed to be stuck at 93% so we lowered the immune suppressant again to see if that would jostle them a bit. They were getting along too well with my remaining "me-cells" so enough of THAT! No more Ms. nice-guy cells...they needed to go at it a bit. May 24th was my 100th day and it was a significant marker because after that day, the possibility of GVHD is much less if there wasn't any during the first 100 days, so that was a good sign for me. I promptly got a cold and a cough and Dr. Bob wanted to see how my own immune system handled it. However, that cough did not improve my singing the following week-end in New Harmony—I told the audience it was my donor's fault—she couldn't hit the high notes evidently—but it was fabulous to be down there and walk the labyrinth at night with dear friends and talk openly about this leukemia thing and not freak out. We have been going to a playwriting conference in New Harmony for at least nine years and our kids have gone there with us every spring. Now they're giant boys and the town seems very small to them. Jack was a baby when we first started there! So that launched us into the hot hot Indiana summer and I went off to the hammock post-haste.

While I was under the maples, hammock-prone, my dear friend Liz, her husband Michael, and their son Nick were heading off to Lake Tahoe that week to ride 100 miles for the Leukemia and Lymphoma Society. What dedication and friendship and love.

During the time at New Harmony, we got word that Allen, the son of Maribeth, the cancer-fighting mom from Chicago, was failing. He had been through a stem cell transplant for Ewing's Sarcoma and had been heroic in his fight for over two years. He had been in and out of the hospital and through so many different treatments. Now it seemed he was having "complications". It was chilling and disheartening and very sad. I had felt so connected with this boy and his family, especially his ever-vigilant mom, and to know that it could all go wrong struck fear in my heart. Tim and I received word few days later that family members were rushing up to Chicago to be with Allen as he was going fast. I wept to think of this brave boy leaving the world, too soon, too soon. I felt the need to hold on—to myself, to my mind, to my cells, lest I be drawn into a dark picture for my own future. It was a strange time, because I felt so much love for their whole family and yet I had to stay away. I could not bring myself to got to the funeral; I thought I might see myself, my own death there and all the terror and sorrow and foreboding might overwhelm me. I felt guilty for that, for thinking of myself, but that is just the way it was and it seemed that Maribeth and her sister Janet both understood. My own news was encouraging, and I tried to focus on life, on the life-force that I could feel building inside of me.

JUNE 4, 2006—The biopsy results are in: NO blasts or any signs of leukemia! Yea! However, my donor cells are hovering around 91% and that is NOT where we want them…we want them to completely get rid of my old cells and be 100% of my blood. Then we can feel more assured that the leukemia will not return. So, it's back to talking to my cells and meditating deep into my bones and helping my own cells say good-bye and the new ones feel strong and dominant! I've been feeling so good and "normal" that I forgot to communicate with my insides…but I need to stay connected for the rest of my life. No slacking off even if it is summertime, and the most beautiful weather these days. I am trying to get the pictures of gardening day on the website…the Gardening Brigade was amazing and continues to help weed and water. The gardens are a visual feast for me. I sit outside and just LOOK and enjoy and TRY not to get my itchy fingers in there to pick that ONE dead flower or ONE weed. I tried to explain to Dr. Bob just what it's like out here in the summer. It's all about the garden and big hayfields and swimming at Liz's lake or the marina and that's it. (Besides driving around to soccer this and soccer that and Connor is in band camp, playing saxophone.) But it's pretty rustic here— last year my sister said it was like camping—but it is just contrary to the way things go here not to dig around in the dirt, go into the barn and feed animals, or swim…but these are things I cannot do for a YEAR!! So, aside from the cough that sounds like a thousand marbles rolling around in the back of a pick- up, I'm feeling pretty good. Tired and achy are par for the course, I guess, and I'm sick of sounding like an old lady chronicling the days aches and pains! I have these words so often in my mind: look to this day, for it is life, the very life of life, for yesterday is already a dream and tomorrow is only a vision— gotta be right here, right now, in the day, in the moment. Love, Jan

JUNE 10, 2006—I saw Dr. Nelson yesterday and it was so up- lifting, for a variety of reasons. First, it had been two weeks and I was suffering from a bit of separation anxiety so it was reassuring just to be there and see everyone, nurses included. I saw a couple of the women who work on the BMT unit, where the transplants happen (as opposed to the clinic where I go for check-ups) and it was wonderful to see them and be healthy and strong. Everyone says how good I look, how healthy. I have to say that I look better than I feel, with all the internal aches and pains in my joints, but Dr. Nelson says that it the result of weaning off the immune suppressant and possibly more en-grafting of donor cells. So he's explaining that they used a dif-ferent procedure to count the cells this past week; instead of from a blood sample, they used marrow from the biopsy and can identify donor cells very easily because they can see the different chromosomes. I'm nodding away as I listen, but then I said, "No. No no no, my donor's chromosomes are female like mine. Right?" He says my donor was a male. I say no, she was a female. 33 years of age and no kids, I remember these details VERY clearly. The nurse says yes, it was a woman, but then she looks in my chart and says no it was a male, 27 yrs old. Now I am outraged and kind of yelling at them: Wait a minute! This changes everything!!! My donor is a MAN!!??? I have to re-think this whole imaginary conversation I've been having with her—ummm, HIM, and I drew a PICTURE of my female donor and me, and NO WONDER the cells are stuck...I've been talking to a woman's cells and they are highly offended! I wasn't really mad, just kind of surprised and actually amused, but they were embarrassed, I think, that I didn't have the cor-rect info. So they all scurried out into the hall and talked to the transplant coordinator, who came back in with a stack of pa-pers. He said my original donor was indeed a woman of 33 with no kids. But the back-up donor was this GUY of 27 and Dr. Nelson liked his "profile" better—whatever that means...they liked it that he was younger as well. SO...that was quite funny to hear about and Tim says that explains the fuzz on my cheeks...ha-ha. So it goes, post-transplant...my body is taking care of this cough, which lingers on and on, but no pneumonia. My bone and joint aches are just part of the whole picture right now, so if it's not scary, I can live with it.

Other news: Liz and her husband Michael and 14 yr. old son Nick came back from their 100 mile ride in Lake Tahoe with flying colors—this was the ride to benefit Leukemia and Lymphoma Society. They said it was intense; all these people riding for cancer patients, survivors and otherwise. They raised a BUNCH of money, which goes toward research and grants to patients—yea Liz! What I loved about it was her ACTIVISM. She is an inspiration to me, and my kids as well.

And finally, yesterday, the Cancer Pavilion at IU Med Center hung 12 of my drawings in the lobby as a beginning to their gallery space. They are trying to incorporate Art into the healing process and into every aspect of the decor. I hope the pictures provide some kind of connection for people going through the cancer/healing journey. I know I craved that connection and art seems to be a good way (non-threatening, non-confrontational) to make it happen. So, all in all, I am reminded that things happen, good and not so good. Another friend has relapsed after two years of remission from leukemia. I can't see the future so I treasure the now moments—I am reminded of this over and over and over. At the hospital yesterday, I saw healthy looking people with no hair and masks on and I saw very sick people, some in wheel chairs with IVs attached to them or gliding by on gurneys, on their way to or from some kind of procedure. It is going on all the time. Thanks and thanks again to the nurses and doctors and researchers and lab techs and cooks and bottle washers etc. at all the hospitals all over the world. I am grateful. Love, Jan

It was actually delightfully funny that my donor was not who I had thought she was. It was a good conversation starter, for sure. It really tickled me; I didn't know if it mattered on any chemical level, but it did matter to me in terms of my visioning, and especially my drawing. The drawings were still so important to me. The very act of it, the feeling of the pencil on the paper, and the colors that would surprise me as I learned to adjust the pressure on the paper, were potent and healing experiences. I never really knew what I was going to draw until I made the first couple of lines. Then I would tilt my head, squint at the paper, bite my lip, mumble maybe, and then it would just flow and turn into a drawing. Sometimes I worked quickly. Other times I drew very slowly, and stopped for a while, only to return to it a day later and have a new perspective. The drawings continued to tell a story that I couldn't tell in words and freed some part of me in the process.

I had become quite a night owl; reading and puttering around into the night and then sleeping late in the morning. This was radically different from the "old" me. My dreams were weird and full of wild images, like large geese that I could ride on, and fields and fields of purple grass that I am walking through. I would toss and turn all night and then sink into a deep sleep in the early morning. So one particular morning, when the dog walked onto the bed and Tim was handing me a cup of coffee, it took me a while to comprehend exactly what he was saying (and why in blazes he was waking me up). "Kelly from IU Med Center called: your cells are 100% donor." The dog was breathing into my face and my eyes were blurry and I was trying to get it... "Your donor cells are 100%...no more YOU in the blood." HOLY COW! I was trying to get some coffee into my system. I said, "Are you sure? Is it true? Are we POSITIVE????" Yes, yes, and yes. So it was a momentous day for me. I felt that something might have been happening because there was a lot going on in my body: cramping hands, aching joints, my swollen gums had totally healed up, my cough was going away and I just felt stronger. The past weekend had been all about soccer—the boys both had the final tournament at home and the World Cup was on and so we were all going strong for three days. And I felt really good, like I could breathe and do stuff—my thinking was not as clear as it used to be but I guess the effects of chemo take a long time to heal. I still couldn't swim for a year and I couldn't garden. My hair was a soft and fuzzy rug on top and silky on the sides, very curly. My skin was extremely sensitive so no tanning, no sun whatsoever. I knew I would have to take a bunch of pills for a long time. But all these things were so minor, so unimportant, so who cares?! I had the feeling my cells finally got the message from all of us to get in there and DO IT because we finally understood who they were and that we respected and loved them! They were moving at the speed of the body and that's a beautiful thing. Blood is amazing. Everything is so relative. There was only room for gratitude and celebration.

Life with all my new cells was interesting and a little weird: I woke up every morning feeling like I was about 110 years old and as the day progressed, I got younger by the hour. Every day brought a new set of body-vibrations to deal with: aches and pains in my joints and muscles, numbness in my hands, and pain at the sites of some past hip biopsies. This was the beginning of a long time of various GVH symptoms and they were very distracting. I just wanted to regain some level of normalcy, even though I knew, intellectually, that "normal" would not be the same normal that I had known. However, just trying to get through the day without focusing on some new body condition was difficult. I felt trapped by my mercurial body, which was changing daily.

I had the opportunity to talk to someone else who has been through her share of hospital experiences, including chemotherapy, and it was so great to talk to someone who knows the weirdness of it all. We were marveling at the fact that we ever went through it; it seemed rather surreal now to remember the hospital and the nurses and doctors who were our constant companions and then the absolute bizarre delayed reaction of, weeks later, having a complete meltdown...after the fact, after the actual trauma of it all...kind of a post-traumatic effect. The whole thing was just miraculous and wonderful and terrible at the same time. I was still walking the tightrope of wondering: am I okay? And then, sometimes, I could slow down and get inside myself a bit and feel the health and the well-being of my cells and my blood, and my heart rate would slow and my blood pressure would drop a bit and all was well in the Land of the Body. It's quite a ride!

Soccer was part of our every waking hour with Jack kicking and juggling out in the back yard and the World Cup keeping us riveted...the Brazil colors were being worn prominently at our house. Connor was getting ready to go to camp on Sunday, off to the world of adventure and smelly shoes at Camp Palowopec. I was reading a lot and drawing and preparing to do the first show of the IRT season, "The Gentleman From Indiana"—a love song to this heartland state for sure. Tim was playing music all over the place and summer was unfolding in a pretty lovely way.

And my garden! The Garden Brigade was coming out to weed and water, helping it all come to fruition. I loved to just stare at it all, pick herbs for dinner, and wait patiently for tomatoes. We were the one-day-at-a-time people. I hoped that was a good thing. I am not sure it will prepare my kids for the working world of their adulthood, but it seemed the only way to get through those days. Maybe slow and steady really DOES win the race? I could only hope so.

JULY 7—Finally had my Dr. Nelson fix today. I was having some serious separation anxiety now that I only see him every three weeks. I was in the waiting area and I thought I recognized another masked face and it was my BMT pal Hannah and it lifted my spirits immeasurably to talk to another traveler on this path. It is bizarre how the language of illness translates from one to another...kind of like a code or secret club. I remember I am not the only one going through the weirdness and that every symptom is as individual as each patient. So my aches and pains and fatigue etc. are just par for the course apparently. I was also part of a round table discussion on family/children services in cancer treatment yesterday and it was IN-TENSE. I had no idea I would be so moved. There were about 15 people who have or have had cancer and I had never been in a room with such a group. There was so much spirit and courage; and this is not an act, this is the real thing. Sometimes talking about it sounds trite or predictable but these are people who have gone through much worse than me, or who had lost someone, or who had not one, but TWO parents with cancer. It was Big, like the weight of it all was palpable and the room was filled with the energy of hope, fear, loss and love. We were asked to recall our diagnosis and how we told our kids, and I had to remember that awful phone call and the fact that I was whisked away to IU Med. and my kids away to friends' houses. It was painful to think about but a relief to see it so far in the past. The new IU Cancer Center building is going up fast and there is great effort to make sure patient services match the beautiful facility. Hooray for asking the right people: the patients. I think there is so much room for art in the healing process and so I am trying to get in my two cents about it. And the really important news is about my hair. Doctor Nelson thought my hair was looking rather "stylish" today but I beg to differ. My hair is so different from last time. It's soft and curly, kind of like a poodle, or a sheep's rear, sort of tawny and gray and ?? I don't think there's an actual word for the color of my hair. So I'm thinking (just thinking, all you purists) about some coloration...maybe red? blonde? platinum? with some organic kind of coloring, of course, like beets. Maybe I'll just brew up a batch and let Tim put it on...mmmm, that would be pretty. I guess it's a very good sign if I can worry about my Hair! and whether to shave my legs! Such trivia is a relief!

July 11, 2006—Doctor Bob prescribed an over-the-counter aspirin; a high dose, coated thing and it's helping with the bone-aches somewhat. It's the numbness and tingling sensations that creep me out. We could deal with it with yet another medication but I want to wait it out for few more weeks and see how it goes. As long as I can hold my coffee cup in the morning and draw by the afternoon, I'm okay. We have a barn full of fresh hay baled from our front field. It seems to me that this is symbolic of our lives going back to a kind of "normal". Summer, until a few years ago, always meant baling hay. Lucas and Tim on the wagon, my father-in-law Lloyd on the ground walking beside the tractor and me driving...this was the picture for many summers. Then Life intervened, in the form of employment (good) and broken machinery (bad) and traveling (good) and illness (bad). Nothing like a little leukemia to keep a family home and tending to the land though, and now we are reaping some of those benefits: a barn full of hay for the horses for the winter and gardens that are endlessly pleasing to stare at and tomato and pepper plants on the verge of fruition. I have never felt so comforted and sustained by our land as I do now.

Finally the Indiana summer really arrived, and so those of us without air conditioning (I think there are three of us in the whole county) were living with ceiling fans and cold showers and cool basements. Needless to say, it slowed me down. But it reminded me of childhood summers. We had no air conditioning then and the summer was a time to eat cold dinners, like fruit salad and sliced cheese and breads. So one day we made pesto with all the basil from the garden and ate cold sliced grilled chicken, crusty French bread and sliced cantaloupe and that was it. No cooking in this heat. My aches were taking on a unique character; moving from my lips and cheeks to my hands and my hips and my neck, in no particular order. I decided it's definitely easier to be really in the sick part of being sick because at least you know what to do. In the transition time, you're wondering: what's next? It is really a kind of limbo full of "what-ifs". You are trying to recover by paying attention to everything that is going on in your body but also trying to be well in that nonchalant way of health. "Where do I stand now?" I was asking myself many times a day, "Am I well?"

I did discuss this "limbo" state with Dr. Bob. It was just so odd to have gotten through the serious stuff and now, in what I was assuming to be recovery, not exactly knowing what to do. I was feeling like my symptoms were mostly too trivial to bring up during the weeks that I didn't actually see Dr. Nelson. But both he and his nurse reiterated that I could—and MUST—call them if I had any concerns. Dr. Nelson said he often wondered how I was doing during the weeks between appointments and I should call him and stay in touch. How about that? Do most doctors do that? I don't know, but I think he's a miracle! I wish he lived next door and we could have him over for dinner or just hang out and have coffee. That whole staff up there was miraculous.

Other breakthroughs: I could do minor gardening with gloves and a mask, I could feed the horses with gloves and a mask, and I could swim in a pool! Holy cow. I was to start rehearsals for IRT's first show of the season on Aug.15 and then I'd be a working girl again. I was slowly, slowly getting back to my life.

JULY 25—It's hot. Really hot. I am happy to say that we don't
have air conditioning so we know just how hot it is!! Nothing
like really FEELING exactly what's going on. Fans and cool
showers and today we'll hang out at the library for a while.
Communal air conditioning centers might be a good concept,
just for a little relief. Has everyone seen "An Inconvenient
Truth"? Anyway, I have been realizing about how this summer
is following a little bit of a pattern from last summer: remission, easing back into work, summer in the hammock, then
this FEELING—like I don't quite know what to do...for example, this website. I do NOT want it to be a blog of my own
ruminations and musings...all of you are creative and brilliant
enough to have your own, I'm sure. But it has been a gathering
of voices and hearts for the purpose of bringing healing and
I'm afraid to let it go. I also remember feeling this way last
summer and then look what happened. The nagging question
of relapse is...well, nagging. It just hovers there in the atmo-
sphere and even in my deepest meditation, when I feel the peace
of just being alive deep in my core, I know that it is shaky. But
I guess that's true all the time. We really don't know what will
happen at any moment so I guess we are all in that dilemma.
It's just that we can't go around worrying about that all the
time or we would be totally dysfunctional. Cancer happens to
give it a very real picture, not some vague wondering. So I guess
all this is a way of saying that I can't give up this website yet,
although I don't feel I have anything more interesting to say
than any of you, and I'm not in crisis at the moment so I don't
have earth-shattering news...so what do we talk about? I love
the community that has sprung up around this whole thing—
My Illness—and I don't want to feel that I own it or am even
responsible for it...it has been an organically evolving organ-
ism, kind of like a beautiful plant that keeps growing and growing. -Jan

Tim and I went to an interesting event: a Bone Marrow Transplant Reunion at a park in Indianapolis on Saturday. There were MANY people there who are survivors and it was remarkable to see all these people who had been through what I'd been through. I also met a woman who was contemplating having a transplant, as her leukemia had some chromosomal anomaly and she was not a good candidate to stay in remission. I talked with her a long time and told her about my experience with it and how fast the recovery process has been going, relative to what we read about. She was so scared about the prospect of it and she was totally amazed by all the survivors. It was so gratifying to be able to offer her encouragement. She kept saying, "If I make it through this..." and I said, "Not IF—you ARE going to make it through this..." And I realized, that from Day 1, everybody at IU Med Center had said, "You WILL make it through this. You WILL win this fight." There was never any doubt and so I just assumed they were right. I think there's something profoundly powerful in that. I also met a man who had his transplant 12 years ago and had met his donor who was a woman much younger than he. He went to her wedding and recently went to visit her with her new baby twins! They are in each other's lives. I SO wanted to meet my donor when the year was up, and even get to know him. Wow, that was an amazing prospect...so much to look forward to.

AUGUST 5, 2006—I saw Dr. Bob yesterday and he said that while I still can't have a cat in the house, I can go swimming!! In a pool or <u>a lake</u>. So I promptly got in the neighbor's pool with the boys and I almost cried. Oh wow, it felt so good to be immersed in water, cool water on a hot day. PLUS, we did races underwater to see who could go the farthest underwater and I almost won. I mean, my stamina was so much better than I thought it would be! And my soccer skills are coming back too; just ask Jack. I guess health is returning and I'm really okay. The Big Difference between now and last year is a TRANS-PLANT!! I have new blood, new life, new cells, so leukemia is out of the picture, as far as I'm concerned. And that is that. Sometimes it feels like the leukemia was a dream. So this is what I'm thinking: the website definitely stays. No, it does NOT remind me of being sick, in fact, it reminds me why I want to be and stay well. It is so great when other people write and say what's going on. And I feel that healing is ongoing so I can still use the help, even though I look and feel "normal". Except for the hair—it's a mass of tiny curls that balloon out around my head like a small, yet burgeoning, cloud. Who knows where they will end? -Jan

The website continued to furnish me with news of the community and I was honored to hear from Maribeth. If I were in her shoes, I might have just crawled under a rock, but she kept in touch and to this day, is working in a hospital dealing with bone marrow transplant patients.

Hi Jan,
Haven't checked in for quite awhile—I'm sure you understand about why that is. Maybe these comments are too serious for here, so I'm sorry for that, but you so eloquently and succinctly struck a chord with your words in your most recent journal entry. You have so brilliantly described all of the phases of the cancer fighting process. I wish I could have had the presence of mind to describe these processes/phases to our friends/family during Allen's fight. Keep fighting; keep writing. -Maribeth

We also heard from Sarah about her family's move from New York City to the country, the gory details of a sinking septic system and the harrowing adventures of actually closing on the place as well as endless tales of her magical son Sam. We all grew to love them and wait for the next installment of their saga. Yes, there was tragedy as well as comedy going on out there. Everybody's stories helped me keep mine in perspective. It was just so good to know that life was plowing ahead, more easily for some than others, but dammit, we just keep going. It is the way of things and all the awareness of it was like nourishing food for me. I just ate it up, all the tales of my friends' lives, and the knowledge that I was in their lives just as they were in mine. No wonder we need art; fiction, opera, theater, painting, on and on; we need to see our lives reflected back to us because it gives us the courage to go on in this crazy, unpredictable life. Tim wrote a song during this time about going to a farmer's barn to buy hay. We were not in any position to bale our own hay that summer and he had to go looking for some. He found this hay farmer tucked between some factories and warehouses, the only farmhouse left in that area. He came home and wrote about the man after talking with him, and the chorus is: "so it goes, so it goes/ you never know what's coming/ might be rain, or wind, or snow/ you wake up in the morning and you bless the things you hold/ never know what's coming, so it goes."

12

Life was indeed up and running. I was cautioned to take it easy, and I really tried. But when you feel well, you want to do the things you've always done. I had so many "mothers" telling me to slow down, to go sit, to rest, rest, rest. Alright, alright! I knew they were right. I needed to conserve my energy because I was going back to work.

THURSDAY, AUGUST 17—It is my third day of rehearsal and it is so fabulous to be back at work. I was worried that I might not be able to hold my own in a room full of creative people having stimulating discussions, but I seem to be able to express myself just fine. I guess not having the distractions of kids, dog, garden, phone calls, dishes in the sink and wondering how my health REALLY is lifts a load off the grey matter and I can actually have ideas and express them. The hour-long car ride up and back is, as always for me, a lovely time to think. I love the uninterrupted time to float from idea to idea and just be with my thoughts. Funny how easy it is to get wrapped up in the business of everyday life once I'm feeling well. I developed a very useful way of meditating to rid myself of stress when I was in hospital, and I try to remember to do that still. But the drive alone, and the full day of work and thinking are energizing and lovely.

We were all at my niece's wedding this past weekend in Michigan. We bought the boys suits for the occasion, and they loved them. Jack wears a suit with élan...with his long yellow hair and his sunglasses; he looked like he was going down the red carpet. On the way to the wedding, Lucas commented that his pinstriped blue suit pants were awfully tight; that he must have gained weight since he had them tailored. Connor had remarked earlier that his pants (also blue pin-striped) were so huge, he was worried they might fall down even with a belt. Suddenly it dawned on me that they might have each other's pants on and it was true. One pair had cuffs, the other not; so they raced in the church to switch pants before the ceremony started. Connor had the honor of walking my sister (mother of the bride) down the aisle so he was panicking to be ready on time. It was like a Marx brothers movie: first they ran one way, and then they ran the other way, and finally found the bathroom where they could change. Connor, of course, looked handsome and confident coming down the aisle, especially since he had the right trousers on!

The reception was fun. I figured I'd dance one or two and watch the rest. But I danced a gazillion times, with all three sons, with Tim, and the bride, and anyone else who would dance. I had so much energy; it felt like the "old days".

On an "interesting" health note, I have some weird sensations in my throat and esophagus that persist, so I am going to have it looked at by a GI guy with a scope next week. I am told that the anesthesia is very specific for this procedure: out like a light and then back to consciousness very quickly afterwards, but I may have no memory of the DAY! So I hope I don't have to learn too much blocking in rehearsal that day...yikes. So life is good. Jack started middle school, now in the same school with Connor, and also on the same soccer team. Such ease of transportation may never come again. I am so grateful for all the help we have had in getting to this point. Thank-you everyone. My gardens, by the way, are bountiful and gorgeous. I love seeing the light change at night. I look forward to really seeing the fall and then the change into winter. I haven't seen a full year of seasons and weather in a long time. Every day is delicious. -Jan

We had to be at IU Med Center at 7:45 to get me prepped for "The Procedure", which entailed a scope going down my esophagus and taking pictures. This is amazing, if you ask me, that a camera is small enough to do that and not rip up your insides. In fact, you feel nothing afterwards, it's a piece of cake. The anesthesia was very interesting. It put me out in a flash and coming out of it was pretty easy. Tim was called into the recovery room and as I was coming to, this is what he wrote down that I said: "They'll have a hard time getting the popcorn out of my car with the picture of the saint in my window." and "After my nap or before it, I would like to do some backward somersaults." AND "What will they do about the chickens in the hallway?" "What chickens?" he asked. "The 6 or 8 black hens that are in the hospital hall." Okay, that was the report from anesthesia-land. And the results of the scope: just a minor infection of some irritated part of my esophagus and medicines could easily take care of it. SO much better than scar tissue or ulcers, which were two of the lovely possibilities. We were much relieved with that diagnosis. I kind of missed the post-treatment days in the hammock but it's hard to make a living in a hammock. I was trying to balance the lessons I learned while I was sick with the beauty of "normal life" and the delight of working, especially in the theater!

Having already reduced my alcohol intake to none, my intake of hot and spicy foods, fruit and vinegary things to NONE, I looked at Dr. Bob with horror when he told me no coffee. "No c-c-coffee???" He said, "Think of the lining of the esophagus like a skinned knee. You wouldn't pour coffee on a skinned knee, would you?" I said, "Yes, I might; if it would perk me up and de-fuzz my brain." He didn't buy it. So I had to eat food in small amounts, many times a day, lots of pasta and greens and cereal and toast. Damn, I thought the days of food problems were over. Otherwise, the bod seemed to be holding up in the post-transplant transition. Dr. Bob said last Friday that in the history of bone marrow transplants, I was the fastest to recover, and that he was thinking of writing a paper about me for a medical journal. I don't know if he was pulling my leg or not. I would have a bone marrow biopsy, the usual for a six-month marker, the following week to monitor the cells and see if I was still all donor.

Six Months!! Sometimes it seemed like it was yesterday and I could still feel the hospital bed, and smell the smells and hear the sounds of the BMT unit. Other times it felt like it was all a dream. I watched a movie called "The Family Stone", which I was advised not to see because of the dying mother theme. I hadn't wanted to see something like that when I was feeling so crummy, but I took a chance and watched it. I completely loved it, loved the characters, loved the whole way the cancer thing was dealt with (subtly and tenderly) and I decided I am in love with Diane Keaton, who is wearing her age with dignity like a badge of honor and still smiles like a girl. So I considered it a turning point, that I could watch a movie about that cancer and dying mothers without collapsing in despair. I was far from despair. Fall was in the air; there was possibility and hope.

Rehearsals for this play consumed my time—we rehearsed afternoons and previewed at night, opened the show on a Friday, did two shows on Saturday, one on Sunday, then finally a day off Monday, during which I recovered from the previous week.

It was time for the six-month bone marrow biopsy. A little Percoset, a little Phenergen and I sailed through the whole procedure. Once again, Tim wrote down what I was saying during the procedure: something about going to Lebanon with Dr. Bob, something about the toxicity of the make-up Kelly was putting on, someone wearing "retirement clothes", and something about the hidden contents of a box I was carrying. I felt great, sleepy, and I don't remember anything about the pain, so I figure that's the way to do it. It was my tenth biopsy since Feb. '05. I imagine my hip bones are riddled with little holes where they've taken samples of marrow. Kelly, Dr. Bob's nurse practitioner and right-hand woman, called with the results: NO Leukemia, and NONE of MY old cells in the blood, ALL DONOR, which is thrilling news. I got that news on the day of opening night, and that made the evening extra sweet. I remembered, when James Still, playwright of "The Gentleman From Indiana" and very dear friend, asked me to do the play, I actually didn't think I could do it. I didn't really know if I would be alive; I really didn't, given all the terrifying info we had gotten about transplants. So it was momentous to be at IRT working. The IRT has been so supportive of me as an artist, and also as a person, during sickness AND wellness. It is a family.

On a more mundane note: my esophagus was healing and I could eat more comfortably, even drink a cup of very milky, tepid coffee. And life in the country was so rich at that time of year; you could just feel the changes daily in the season. The sounds of crickets and peepers were slowing down, fireflies were having a hard time at night in the cool, damp air so they laid in the grass and flickered, and the horses were happy the flies were disappearing. The horses got out of their fence one night and Tim and I had to herd them into their paddock with flashlights and cans of grain. The next day we had a message on our answering machine from a neighbor on the other side of our back field, telling us she had a cow in her back yard and was it ours? Apparently lots of animals were restless in the changing weather and were looking outside their enclosures for more goodies. Who says country life isn't interesting?

OCTOBER 2—I happened to go by the BMT clinic a week and a half ago to pass out some info about the play, and saw Dr. Bob in the hallway. He wondered what I was doing there and I told him. He asked if I had a few minutes to go across the hall to the hospital unit, where I had stayed in February for the transplant itself, to see the nurses and show them a "well person"! Seems they had a rough morning (I didn't ask the details) but a couple of the nurses were feeling very low and had told the doctor that "they see patients when they're sick and when they die, but not when they're WELL". So I went over as a sort of ambassador of health. Everybody was great, and happy to see me, and so excited for me about the play and just my general state of health. I look so different from when they had last seen me: about 15 pounds heavier and with some hair...it was good for them to see that people really do get well, and so good for me to be there and not be sick. Then I went to 5-N, where I had been last year when I was first diagnosed and I saw doctors and nurses I hadn't seen in over a year. It was surreal to be there; even the pattern of the linoleum tiles was familiar, as I had walked those hallways so many times, with nothing to look at but the patterns on the floor. It was astonishing to be there as a healthy person. Then I saw Mary, who had been one of my primary nurses and I started to cry. She was an absolute rock for me, even stayed after her shift was over once because I was going through a rough time and she wanted to stay until I was stable. And the first time I left the hospital to go home, after 30 days, she was the one I was most afraid of being away from. She knew it and was so reassuring that I would be okay, and of course, I believed her because she always was straight with me. She is a living angel. So it seems that my cells are behaving well and doing their appointed jobs. I talk to them still and I feel a wave of calm when I do. I am taking care of myself like a recovering person, but also feeling the joy of "normal" life (if there is such a thing). I know I am not out of the woods, that it takes years to get back all the energy, and maybe the thought of recurrence never really goes away, but right now life is good. I'm trying to stay there, in that NOW. -Jan

OCTOBER 14—I saw Dr. Bob on Thursday and he said I have an abundance (actually, over-abundance) of eosinophils. Isn't that a great word? Pronounced eeyo-sin-o-fills. They are the white blood cells responsible for keeping the worm population under control—did you know we all have microscopic worms in us? The thing of it is that my immune system is doing a balancing act and will be for years, so the docs monitor what's going on and adjust meds etc. accordingly. At least the immune system is functioning! I had been having aches and pains in my bones again, and was happy to know it was those pesky eosinophils and not a relapse. So I am taking a tiny dosage of prednisone again, which has done the trick in terms of aches and pains, but my face is a tad puffy. F'gahdsake, I tell you, if it's not one thing it's another. I have to remind myself that all this is far better than returning to the hospital or undergoing chemo, so I am really trying to be gracious about it. But secretly, in my deepest darkest self, I am SICK of it and I just want to be normal and not puffy and spotty and taking loads of pills. So there. That said, I'm happy as a pig in mud, because I am painting our empty bedroom. It will be my drawing/writing room and it is turning out to be the room of my dreams. I have literally dreamt of this room for about 10 years, ever since the first time Tim and I went to New Harmony and saw a little garden shed painted with lovely colors so I just decided to DO IT and it is really great.

One thing leukemia has done for me has been to ask the question "why wait?" and "why not?" It is so easy to think the unorthodox and exciting things and plan to do them someday. But I am really feeling and needing to say NOW, do it now, don't wait, take a step...even if it's painting a room in wacky colors. Such as: one wall is lavender, one is mossy green and the other is rose-pink, with butter yellow trim. Oh it's luscious and I am anxious to get in it with my table and chair and start working.

This was a time of great introspection for me. I was dealing with health issues that seemed fairly trivial compared to the big disease called Leukemia, but on the other hand, they inhabited my body and that is, after all, where I live. That idea of the body as my "home" reminded me of a realization I had when I was about six or seven years old. I was sitting out in our backyard in the grass, and I was looking at my bare legs and feet, which were sticking straight out in front of me. I marveled at the fact that my toes were so far away from my head, and yet that was still me too. My body, which I could see out in front of me, was me. I had been thinking the real "me" was deep inside my head, and the rest of the body was like baggage.

I also remember a movie where a woman, who is noticing a guy riveted on her breasts, says, "Hey! I'm up here!" meaning for him to look at her eyes. Where are we, exactly? Are we in the whole of our body? Or are we spirit riding around in the body? I think both. But I am aware of how much our body is who we are, for the health of it, the very chemistry and physiology, is intertwined with thoughts and feelings and there really is no separation.

I was aware of the dichotomy of having the knowledge of the preciousness of every single moment, and also trying to live in the regularity of daily life. I know a few other people who have faced near-death experiences and to go on living in the real world, the "normal" world, is a challenge. Reconciling the two realities is a challenge. And not falling apart over the whole thing is a challenge. Many days were fraught with nagging questions and angst. And my inner dialogues were not all that comforting.

One night at a friend's dinner party, I was kind of wandering around outside, not feeling very sociable, when a woman approached me. She reminded me that she had written about my transplant for a Bloomington magazine. She said, "I remember you saying that you talked to your bones. Do you still do that? I thought that was so cool." Well, you could have knocked me over with a feather. NO, I wasn't doing that, in fact, I wasn't doing anything remotely like that. I had slipped unknowingly into complacency and was just going along like my body should be serving me, not me serving my body. I looked at her with surprise, and said "no!" but I thanked her profusely for reminding me to do so. How easily we forget and take things for granted.

The Graft versus Host condition moved to my mouth and I had sores and a feeling like my tongue was sunburned. Not exactly conducive to fine dining, and that of course, was hard for me, foodie that I am. It hurt to swallow and to talk and I wasn't planning to stop either of those activities in the near future so I had to tough it out. I started on prednisone to ease the inflammation, and that in turn, made me a bit nutty. I felt like I could scrub floors and cook for 100 plus eat my weight in persimmon pudding, which unfortunately, I had made in almost such a quantity. I had put the 11x13 pan of the butter and cream rich pudding in the refrigerator. Since I was working at the computer in the office 10 steps away, I would walk into the kitchen, pull back the foil just enough to spoon out a few bites, and then back to work. Imagine my surprise when I pulled back the cover and there was none left! My steroid-addled appetite had no "off" button and I was just shoveling it in. The only comforting factor of the GVH was the leukemia-fighting component. In other words, if the cells were that active, they would be equally active against cancer cells. So the GVH had a trade-off.

Around this time, my friend Carol came up with a very interesting travel plan that she envisioned, and it involved me. She has family in London, and also had a daughter studying abroad for a year in the south of France and she thought <u>we</u> should go on a trip to visit them. I couldn't quite imagine it. I asked Dr. Bob if I could possibly do such a thing, fully expecting him to say no. He thought it was a fine idea and that if my blood levels remained constant, I would be fine. Yikes! I might really go to Europe. Then came the issue of financing the trip. Carol had found amazing prices on flights and we had to decide fast. A residual check arrived in the mail from one of the movies Tim had done years before and it would more than cover the trip. So what was holding me back? I realized I was scared to be so far away, "what ifs" lurking in my brain. Dr. Bob assured me he was a phone call away and I should feel good about going. Then I had that instinctual feeling—the one that says "do it now, who knows what will happen, when you will get this opportunity again, who knows if you'll be alive—no one knows, so just GO"

So we did. We flew first to London and stayed right in the center of the city with Carol's aunt. London! It was so amazing to be there and we had the sunniest, most beautiful weather. I was definitely moving slower than in the old days, and I did feel like the invalid of the group, but they adjusted to my speed and off we went. We saw much of the city, but the place that I think I loved the most was the Tate Modern art museum. First of all, the admission is free, so everybody hangs out there; kids, teens, families, punks, goths, pink-haired and tattooed street performers, and blue-haired grandmas…you name it, everyone was there. And I also remembered how much I love to be in a room full of art. Just to stand there, and look at these works that I had studied in art history class, and the modern work that I really loved…it was breathtaking. It made me think of home and why didn't I go to the museums there? I know the Tate is extraordinary, but standing in a room full of art can happen in Indiana too, and I made a mental note to make sure to do that when I got home.

Then we flew to Marseilles, to meet Carol's daughter Anna, and we took the bus to Aix, where she was living. We spent most of our days walking around the charming city. Because it was December, Christmas decorations were abundant and we saw the place where they make the "santons" the clay figures that are set up in a village setting, with all the figures of the town, as well as baby Jesus and the usual crèche figures. So you might have the baker, the farmer, and the butcher as well as shepherds and the more familiar figures of the Nativity scene. We were totally hooked and brought home many "santons". We also went to Cezanne's atelier, his studio, and marveled at the fact that some of his things were still there, arranged just as he might have had them. We saw the views out his window, just as he had seen them, as well as the light, an extraordinary element in his paintings. That light was the light he saw. The mountain that we could see was the mountain he painted, and the luminous countryside was his also. Everything astonished me.

We ate amazing food in Aix, whether it was at a simple café or being feted by Anna's friends who hosted a six-course meal that makes my mouth water just thinking about it. Foie gras, roast duck, pates, crusty breads, and tossed greens with vinaigrette; mmmm, it was a celebration of food.

But I was becoming somewhat fatigued as the trip went on, and I had to slow my pace down. I was also getting a bit round in the face as well as developing some swelling in my legs. I chalked it up to the astounding amounts of Stilton cheese that Carol and I had consumed in London. Or maybe it was the crepes au chocolat that we loved in "our crepe place" under the street in Aix. As our trip finished up, I had a little cough and I wore my mask all the way home on the plane. When I returned home, I had a "cold" but I was feeling okay.

DECEMBER 21—I think we will keep this website alive until February 14, the anniversary of the transplant and then sign off. It seems symbolic to do so. I look forward to meeting my donor, if he will agree to that. I look forward to thinking about leukemia less and less each day, although I plan to do some kind of work for bone marrow/ stem cell donation awareness, and then....who knows? Many doors have opened since leukemia came my way and we'll see.... xxoo -Jan

13

Well. Even the best laid plans… I was recovering from my "little cough", and then family and friends descended on the home for the holidays, and everyone that arrived was sick! I'd have to say it was "denial" that made me think it was okay for me to be close with everyone and not worry about my own cough. The cough turned into something more, something that felt suspiciously like pneumonia. I tried to avert it, but when I couldn't sleep for coughing and wheezing, I knew…the jig was up. On Dec. 30 I called the BMT doctor on call, some resident I had never met, and he said the only way to come in at night was through the emergency room, and I did NOT want to do that. I felt that I was an alum of sorts of IU Med Center and I deserved special treatment. I don't know whether that was logical thinking or just uppity, but I could not imagine myself going into that hospital, where I had spent close to 90 days and nights, as a "regular customer". I couldn't imagine being an unknown commodity in the emergency room, after all I had been through. So I waited until the next morning and I called the nurses station in the BMT and begged them to find me a place to stay. I knew there were two outpatient rooms that could be used as overnight rooms if necessary and I asked for that. They were all kind enough to let me stay there, with nurses I knew, and a more reasonable room. Otherwise, I would have been in the old area where I first was admitted, and I thought that would just be too depressing. I was unsure about being "demanding" but I felt my well-being depended on it.

I was in for two days, getting massive antibiotics and sleeping most of the time. I was absolutely exhausted. A sputum sample was sent to the lab and it was discovered that I had RSV, Respiratory Synsasial Virus, something usually found in babies…and transplant patients! I came home January 1, 2007.

I was home back on the couch and feeling like I was recovering from a cold. One day I roused myself and drove the kids to school whereupon I quickly became exhausted. When the nurse called from the hospital that day to ask follow-up questions and make sure I was all right, I asked, "So what exactly am I supposed to do after pneumonia?" She said I needed to stay at home, not go anywhere for two weeks at least, rest, drink lots of water, and take my meds. Well! Another mandate to do nothing! I complied with pleasure—doctor's orders, after all. I read and ate and rested. After about five days of this, I decided to go up to my special pink and lavender room and poke around. I saw some old drawings and my journals scattered about my desk. I thumbed through a journal and smiled to myself as I remembered the "old days" in the hospital. I thought, "I really should start writing about this whole experience." I remembered, when I was first diagnosed, trying to find something about leukemia in every bookstore I happened to go into, and there were stories of all kinds of cancers, but not leukemia. So I walked around my room some more and wondered how to begin. I thought I better go down and wash some dishes. Then I thought maybe I should walk the dog. Then I came back up and strolled around my room. After about three days of patrolling the house and perusing my desk, I finally just sat down and started to remember and then I started to write.

JANUARY 7, 2007—Okay, I think I am lucid enough to write…anyway, it was unreal to be in the hospital again and on New Years Eve!! How ridiculous. The whole thing totally depressed me for a couple of days and I looked ahead to 2007 wondering what the hell am I going to do? I feel like this whole chemo/transplant thing has aged me far ahead of my time. I am voicing complaints appropriate for a woman 20 year older than me! My joints, my lumps and bumps, my skin, my hearing…what? WHAT?? Oy vey etc. etc. So I am heading into this year with many questions. I feel I am thigh deep in the muck of post-transplant weirdness, so it's not a big surprise, at least. Insurance will be the Big Question this year, as I have lost qualification for one insurance, which covered everything from the beginning, and will start a Cobra co-pay. This will be the subject of much study in the weeks to come.

Have I mentioned my EYES? My PUFFY eyes? Some days it looks like I have been punched in the eyeballs, splotchy and swollen, and then my face developed a sort of thin crust all over, that soaked up emollients and lotions as fast as I could put them on. So a little cortisone cream seems to have quieted that down. Why is it that a steroid can take care of EVERYTHING??? I was prescribed prednisone for my cough, and I refused to fill the prescription. Dr. Bob said okay, but if I start "coughing my head off" (his technical term) I should reconsider. But I swear, every time some swelling or inflammation comes, boom, let's throw a steroid at it. It seems to be a medicine with as many side effects as benefits. I guess when I was looking leukemia in the eyeball and wondering about the fatal effects of transplants, I wasn't too concerned about the aches and pains I'd heard about post-transplant. At that point, who cares? But human nature being what it is, one's perspective changes and now the whole picture looks different. It's a different kind of challenge. I never, in a million years, thought I would be one of those "sick people", with aches and pains and complaints. And now, here I am, kvetching with the best of them. xxoo -Jan

Dr. Bob called me at home on a Saturday to see how I was feeling and to discuss the prednisone dosage with me, knowing that I was not keen to be on steroids for an extended period of time. I was not happy with the round face or the jittery way I felt sometimes, but he said not to fret, that it is not a bad thing, just an inconvenient thing. Though hearing him explain that it would be a short but intensified dose, and the fact that he would call me every couple of days to see how I'm doing, reassured me. So I was the Prednisone Girl once again and I hoped to keep my appetite under some control this time.

The other development was that I signed a waiver sheet releasing my contact information to my donor and started that process of meeting him, if he would be willing to do so. He would get the same waiver to sign on his end from the Bone Marrow Registry and we had to wait and see. So I decided not to end the website on 2/14 like I had thought because I thought the meeting with the donor might be a cool thing to share with everyone. Instead, I suggested we all should party in all parts of the globe and celebrate health and life in general. I wrote:

> Valentine's Day has never been so sweet. It's only a month away. Get your pinks and reds out and get ready to party!!! Kiss all the people you love! love love love -Jan

Dr. Bob called frequently to check on my symptoms and monitor the prednisone. He said I needed to listen to my body and I should be able to tell if I need to go up to three Preds or stay at two...he said, of course, to call if anything's weird but we'd would talk at the next appointment after he's looked at blood labs. So it was sinking in: this is post-transplant reality. Dr. Bob referred to it as my "funny little GVH". I said, "Oh yeah, real funny." He said it was a tad unusual but that we had to train the new cells to settle down. I asked if they were trainable, and he said "Yes indeed". I believed him. He's so smart, this guy, and so thoughtful. I was, and am, around the bend for him, clearly.

The cold weather was a bit much for my post-transplant self. I was already dreaming of spring. I remembered last spring as one of the most beautiful ever. I remembered the sounds of songbirds and lots of green, which I was longing for.

FEBRUARY 1, 2007—So much for thoughts of spring...this is finally winter! Some snow on the ground and the temperature is in the teens, plus today is sunny and blue-blue sky so it is amazingly beautiful. Tim and I sang in Michigan over the past weekend and it was very cool to be onstage again, a little less sure of my voice (post-pneumonia scratchiness) than I'd like to be, but I found my groove about halfway into the first set! My one-year anniversary is fast approaching...February 14 is The

Day and it is exciting to think about it. I remember being in the hospital and it was hard to imagine a whole year from then...seemed like forever. And now it's here. I have been going back through the journal and guestbook—it has been so intense to look back and see what we all went through, how you all stayed with the process, checking in and sending thoughts and prayers and love and jokes and poems. I just get overwhelmed as I read and remember. I had forgotten about a lot of it, blissfully, I suppose...I had forgotten some of the difficult times of the chemo and I had forgotten how bad it was. But now, from this vantage point of a year of recovery and healing, I find it rather exciting (in a weird sort of way) to realize what I went through. And so did you all. We got through it together. Love, Jan

February 10, 2007—Okay, it's getting closer to the Big Day, which I'm sure will be anti-climactic...kind of like the transplant itself. I remember thinking that a year seemed like so far away last February, and now it seems to have gone by so fast. I am feeling the GVH in new ways all the time. This week it's the skin on my back and neck and face: feels like I have a bad sunburn or something. I am still on a tiny dose of cortisone as well as all the other meds, but relative to liver failure or something like that, I guess I'm doing pretty well. As a folksinger friend of ours says: "At least I'm on the right side of the dirt." I see Dr. Bob on the 20th to review my "status", maybe have a bone marrow biopsy, and go from there. He called me at home a couple of nights ago—which is so thoughtful and wonderful, I might add—and he wanted to know how I was doing since he only sees me once a month now and he knew I wanted to explore the idea of visiting my sisters in Florida. He said he'd prefer that I NOT travel right now, wants me to be completely without cough. So I am disappointed not to be able to see them on my birthday, which we've been trying to do for three years. I am waiting to hear from the Bone Marrow Registry and my donor. We'll know next week if he would like to meet me, and how and when.

The snow almost feels dry it's so cold. I can't get enough of looking at the bare branches against the open sky; they never ceases to amaze. -Jan

WEDNESDAY, FEBRUARY 14, 2007—OKAY, IT'S HERE... I AM ONE YEAR OLD TODAY, IN A MANNER OF SPEAK-ING... THE ONE YEAR ANNIVERSARY OF THE TRANSPLANT. IT IS A BEAUTIFUL DAY AFTER A SLEET STORM AND ALL THE TREES ARE COV-ERED IN SPARKLY ICE. I AM IN BED WITH A COLD THAT I AM TRYING TO STEER AWAY FROM PNEU-MONIA. AGAIN. SO IT'S ALL DAY UNDER THE COV-ERS WITH TISSUES, TEA, THIS COMPUTER AND MANY NEW YORKER MAGAZINES. I WILL KEEP YOU POSTED ON THE PROCESS OF MEETING MY DONOR... WE SHOULD KNOW SOON IF HE IS WILLING TO MEET. THIS IS A VERY SWEET VALENTINE'S DAY. LOVE, JAN
P.S. what is the difference between uploading and download-ing? really.

Still no news about the donor. I was at IU Med Center for my appointment and inquired; everyone there is excited thinking about our meeting. The transplant coordinator sent a message again through the BMT registry and so we would wait and see. I was there for a routine check-up and found a few interesting aspects of my post-transplant days. First of all, my head cold was still lingering, and Dr. Bob said it could be there for some time. My immune system was slow to ramp up and by the time it's raring to go, the baddies (the bacteria or virus) are gaining in strength, so the whole process of getting over the cold would take longer. Also, I was having some interesting bruising and "crust-like" appearance around my eyes. There was some level of GVH wreaking very slight havoc with my skin, so I went up to the dermatologist on the 3rd floor and had a skin biopsy (this would be my fourth of such a procedure). The treatment was an extra-strength cream that he wanted me to use anyway, so the biopsy was just to verify what exactly was going on. As always, they took a picture. I swear, my grandkids are going to open their biology books one day and say "I know her!" as I am laid out on the pages of their text book as an example of some horrific looking skin condition.

Feb. 21 is my real birthday. You are all presents, the best ever, and I thank you for everything. Sandy from Minnesota (you know that name from the website) sent me a most excellent gift today: a compilation of all the poems Mary had put on the site. I made the boys read some out loud tonight at the dinner table, and then Tim read a couple, and I read one. It was so fun, and funny, because when I was growing up, my dad made us give speeches to each other at the birthday dinner table. We loathed it at the time, but I think it wasn't so bad, and we laugh hysterically about it now. So here I was, repeating a loose version of that old ritual tonight with the guys. They thought it was "dumb". I thought it was heaven.

FEBRUARY 23, 2007—Life is on the Move! I've had to get up from the computer twice to go out and see the Sandhill cranes that are trilling and circling overhead. They fly very high but their song is so distinctive. It is miraculous to see them all up there doing their thing.
A CT scan showed the mother of all sinus infections residing in every nook and cranny of my head, so I'm on some very fancy (and pricey) meds for at least a month. Also, the skin biopsy came back as a "yes" to GVH, level 2. I forgot to ask how many levels there are...I guess that could be bad if there was level one, and level two, ba-boom. So I need some serious cream slathered all over my back and shoulders three times a day, and a different ointment on my face, which continues to crustify—new word. Tim and the boys and even my father-in-law have had to administer the cream since it's on my back, which I can't reach so well. Last night, as Tim is out of town, I asked the boys to do it. Jack volunteered but when he saw the stitches on my shoulder from my biopsy, he almost barfed and had to call Connor in to do it. Connor, ever the cool one, had no problem with stitches or spotty skin and doctored me up.

Life goes on with the teens. Jack is 13 this coming March 11. Yikes!

AND, I got word from my donor: he is happy to know I am doing well but chooses to remain <u>anonymous.</u>

 <u>ANONYMOUS!?</u>

I had been napping when the BMT coordinator called with that info but it didn't sink in until today and I am really disappointed. It seemed like it would be such a cool ending to the story. What am I thinking? "End" to my story? The story goes on and on, whether we meet Mr. Wonderful or not. Now I can make up some fictional character—you know, for when the movie comes out, or when we talk about him. I mean, HE won't know, right? So he can be Brad Pitt...omigod, maybe it IS Brad and he IS famous and he doesn't want to go public with this. Oh well... I am writing a journal about all of this and it is just one more funny twist in the story. From your crusty (like a good baguette) friend with love, Jan

14

April 2007 and spring really was around the corner. Again. I love how that happens. One more trip around the sun, and there I was, back in the spring, but a different spring. Not a spring in the hospital. Not a spring hiding indoors, only to walk outside with a mask. This was a spring of a new me.

One of those spring days, I was out in the garden poking around, having Connor help me chop up the dirt and hoe it and rake it and get it ready to plant a few rows of lettuce, radishes, and spinach. I hadn't planted my own garden since the spring of 2004. And, as it was spring in Indiana, the weather was changing almost hourly. The soil was soaking up the sun, and then there would be a torrential rainstorm or a couple of hours of banging winds with branches crashing to the ground, then a cold frosty morning which melted into 70 degrees by the afternoon. It was spring again, just as it had been in this part of the country for hundreds of years; people tilling and planting just like me, for hundreds of years.

Yet the Spring of my Body was a new one. Never had there been a spring like this; never had these cells been growing in my body and nurturing me and wreaking havoc occasionally and generally keeping me on my toes.

I made peace with the notion of a mysterious donor, a young man out there who has his own reasons for staying anonymous. But I still send him blessings, and so do all my family and my friends, and so do my doctors and nurses. Does he know what he has done? Does he know what gratitude is floating around in the world for him?

I was walking down our long gravel lane the other day, ruminating on the news that my "Donor-Guy" would stay a mystery, and I thought, "Well, of course. He was 27 years old, now 28, he's so young. He doesn't want some middle-aged woman falling apart with gratitude all over him, he wants to protect himself. Also, what if something were to happen to me? He might feel terribly guilty, so he just chooses to remain in the shadows. My vision of meeting him and hugging and being in each other's lives is just MY fantasy and he's got his own life to live." And that's all right with me.

I felt good; a quiet elation came over me. To know anything is fairly wondrous anyway. I seem to just walk around with questions begetting more questions and I'm in a muddle a lot of the time. This was true even before chemo-brain. But it's not an unpleasant muddle. Rather, it's a kind of agreement with the universe that says: Okay, there's so much going on that I don't understand, but still I will keep trying. Trying to make a "good" life, whatever that is. Trying to see the light when there is darkness all around. Trying to pass on my love of this life to my children, to let them know that it is worth it; after all the anguish and all the pain and all the confusion, even after all that, it is worth it to live this life. With or without leukemia, with or without illness, with or without challenges, this life is IT. It is all we know, it is all we have, and come what may, it is ours to do with what we will.

As I write now, I am in the throes of different GVH problems. I have developed hyperglycemia from the steroids, which in turn has triggered my cholesterol to shoot up. The cholesterol medicine caused some muscle atrophy in my legs and I was "jelly-knees" for a while. I am shooting insulin three times a day like a pro, hoping this is a temporary condition until I am off steroids. My skin is pretty ravaged, mottled and puckered. I have some extreme pain in my hips that may require cortisone shots and eventually, surgery. I still need to stay away from large groups of people, such as schools or malls, as my immune system is still quite compromised. I get physically exhausted easily, but I try to take a walk everyday. I have a condition called schleroderma, which is an inflammation and thickening of the tissue beneath the skin, and it is especially prominent on my abdomen and hips. It feels like I am wearing a lead belt around my waist—

not so fun. And I am on antibiotics and anti-inflammatory meds and immune suppressors and…whew! The list goes on.

I had to drop out of a play at the IRT because I could not handle the physical aspects of it. I was to play Gertrude in "Hamlet" and, as his mother, I would have to be thrown to the ground when they argue. Back in the day, as they say, I would have loved that! But I will not be acting or teaching for a while, not until I get my strength back. I think this time is particularly difficult because I was prepared to be "well"—so I compare myself with well people. When I had leukemia, I compared myself to people with cancer and I came up way ahead of the pack. Now, by comparison, I seem disabled. The things that have always located me in the world are not available to me now: work, volunteering, running with the kids, eating lots of good food, exercising and just being on the move. It is a time to redefine myself, but I don't always *want* to. It is a struggle, and I am reminded of how I was more comfortable being introspective and meditative when I was really sick. Maybe I can get some of that inner peace back by slowing down, being in the moment. Hmmm, easier said than done. I get that "monkey mind" like the Buddhists say, and I'm off to the races with wondering and worrying. I should know better by now, but it is an endless lesson for me, apparently. A friend of mine wrote me that I didn't have to DO things to be valuable, I just had to BE. Part of me sneered at that, "Hah, no way! Of course, I have to <u>do</u> things to be of value; I have to show the world who I am and that I <u>can</u> do all these things." But right now, I absolutely, physically, cannot be a do-er. I am an observer, a contemplater, a quiet thinker. I'm a little bit like a hermit, staying at home so much so I don't get sick out there in germ world.

Tim continues to be a rock and amazes me with his domestic prowess. He has become a chef, a chauffeur, an organizer of all things soccer and school, a sounding board for the boys, along with his usual skill at doing dishes and laundry, two of his favorite tasks. I know it has to be hard for him, though, to look at me and see my disease, or rather the effects of its treatment, written all over my face and body, like a map. I hardly recognize myself in the mirror; what must it be like for him? I have days of low energy, fatigue and exhaustion and I have days of ebullience. I have to push myself to keep going, even though I might be sick of it, push myself to walk and stretch, fighting against the inevitable effects of steroids.

Connor and Jack watch me, look at my wispy hair or the puckered, lumpy skin on my legs and I think they have to wonder: "is she always going to be like this?" Do they even remember the old me, the mom with long blonde hair and high, wide cheekbones and a big, toothy smile? Do they remember that I used to race mountain bikes or chase them to the soccer ball or hit a softball way out into our front field? Do they remember that I used to run; that I loved to just flat-out run? I doubt it. And yet, for all the looking at me I think they're doing, they are remarkably un-judgmental. One day I said I felt self-conscious about going to a soccer game with my round face and bumpy skin, and Connor said, "Mom, you look fine. Don't worry about it." I don't think he was just trying to make me feel better—it's really how he sees me. Jack, too, said he didn't think I looked that different. I guess because they see me all the time, and I look in the mirror only occasionally, I surprise myself more than them. And they are more forgiving as well.

Much has transpired for both boys since I began writing this memoir. Connor's focus is on music; listening to it, playing it, and writing. He is following in our footsteps in a way, the path of an artistic life. I can't exactly tell him not to; it's what we do. But it's a hard life, as he has seen. All of my kids have seen the highs and lows of following an artistic vision, a life full of rejection and disappointment, as well as the highs of having self-expression validated by audiences or readers or viewers. But it is worth it—to be able to do what you love and to create is truly a remarkable life. (Paying the bills just doesn't always fit into the picture!) He plays on his high school soccer team and he distinguishes himself nicely. He doesn't have the rabid competitiveness of his younger brother, but he does what needs to be done when he's on the field. He seems to have found a niche and a level of inner comfort, as if he likes being in his own skin. He's very tall, in fact he towers over me at 6'3" (I have shrunken to 5'7") and there are times when I feel powerless as we venture into an inane argument over messy rooms or the whereabouts of his cell phone.

But I don't get as distraught as I did when Lucas and I would battle in his high school years. I was truly worried and anxious during those arguments, fearing that every sign, positive or negative, had tremendous meaning for his adult life. Now I see that people, my own children especially, are on their own paths, and messy rooms, although they do need to be cleaned up, are just not that important.

Jack is a Math whiz in a way that none of us could have imagined. He's a music hound also, and when he told us that he had to give up guitar lessons because he had so much algebra homework, I was tempted to tell him to quit the extra math class instead. (Tim advised me against this.) Where did he come from, this kid? None of the rest of us has this math-brain. Tim and I are both intrigued and pleased by it, and now that he can drive, he can get himself to his 6 a.m. calculus work sessions. He and Connor attend different high schools and each of them is in the school that suits them best.

Lucas is working away, up in Chicago, after undertaking his Big Trip. He traveled throughout Mexico and Central America for four months, staying with people through a network called "Couch Surfing". He is fluent in Spanish and wrote a blog to keep us all informed of his travels and especially of the different foods he was trying. He's quite a foodie, and a lovely writer, as it turns out. We'll see where all that takes him.

So the family carries on. The disease is woven into the fabric of our beings in varying degrees. Leukemia has given to us all, and it has taken away. It is part of us in hidden ways as individuals, and it is part of our collective self, as a Family. Just like all the things that ever befall us, I suppose, but Cancer is a profound visitor in one's life. I don't know how this experience will influence my children's lives as they make choices, as they learn, and work, and travel. But it is in us all, no question.

I still have moments, like the ones when I was first home after chemotherapy and my world seemed to have turned inside out. I can be in the room with someone, a family member or a friend, and I can see us framed by a bigger picture, like having one foot in the Great Unknown and the other in the kitchen. I can feel the greatness and the absolute smallness of our lives. It's like having a vision, even though

I know it is only just the room and me and the people in it, but it's profound. We are amazing, just being in our skins, and we are all so beautiful in our sweet little human ways. I feel a big love emanate from inside me and I think I can see the whole panorama of birth, life, and death all around all of us. It feels like The Big Picture. We are so lucky to have each other; anybody, in any way, to be able to be together on this planet for the short time we are here.

Of course, I don't go around talking like this all the time. We just get into the life we are given and we ride along on the river of days. But every once in a while, it's good to share this secret, this little bit of insight that comes with a serious illness or a near-death disaster. Then, we blink, take a couple of breaths, and carry on.

But with all my post-transplant ailments, I can still draw, and I can still write. I can go for walks and socialize in small groups of people, like having my girlfriends over for coffee. I am continually looking for ways to delve into this mysterious road we are all traveling. Making art continues to comfort me and stretch my mind. In fact, I have ventured out of the world of colored pencils and on to pastels and watercolors, looking ahead to painting maybe one day on a big canvas! Some wild ideas for paintings are brewing in my head. I really do believe we all have it within us to express our unique vision of the journey we are on and it seems to be a healing thing. At least for me, the creative, artistic path is an essential thing. It was part of my healing, and it is part of the life ahead.

So the story doesn't have a nice tidy ending with a picture of me hugging my donor. Nor does it end with any surety of continued remission. It is a never-ending story, because no matter what happens to me, there will be someone else who comes after me and has leukemia and will go through whatever treatment is offered at that time, and she will follow in her own path, and then onward from there. All I can say is, I hope she can ask for support and receive it; receive all the love that is given to her, and all the healing and nurturing; that she can be open to the healing and to the love that will be coming her way, even though she may not recognize it at first.

Cancer is so prevalent these days. Certainly my own eyes have been opened by my experience of it, but I now see it everywhere. Part of that is my age; part of it is the age we live in. Treatments are becoming more sophisticated, more specific, less harrowing. But the disease itself shows no signs of abating. It is unlike no other illness – it is not a bacteria or a virus or a parasite. It is the deep chaos of the genetic material in the cells—our own cells gone awry. Why? Why? No less than an earthquake of my soul, leukemia shook me up—turned me inside out and back again. It drew back any veils that time had pulled over my deepest self and revealed that self, once again, to me. It permitted me to speak things I had grown away from. Oddly enough, it gave me new life.

I sometimes wonder, in this post-transplant time with its ups and downs, what I might never do again. Will I ride a horse ever again? Will I ever go on a roller coaster? Will I play soccer again with my sons? Will I walk the endless blocks of my favorite city or hike the hills of our back fields? I don't know. My "health", relative to the old me, is uncertain. But relative to life itself, I'm a winner. I am aware. And I'm vertical! And I am grateful.

One of the soccer parents once questioned me, while we were waiting for a game to begin, about the main lesson I had learned from the whole "leukemia-thing" as he called it. And I replied without hesitation: "Gratitude." My life is now one of gratitude. It is not something I have to work hard at; it is just something I walk around with, inside. You could say it's in my bones. I once read somewhere that gratitude is not a natural human emotion. It has to be taught. I have had many teachers over the years, demanding and challenging experiences that have shaped me, but none so powerful as my beautiful leukemia.

Afterword
And "How to be a Patient"

Another year has passed since I began writing about this journey through leukemia and stem cell transplant. My perspective has changed, again, especially since I have had so many health issues to contend with. It is much easier to be in the hospital when everyone is taking care of you and keeping records and charts and bringing food and clean jammies. Now I am in charge, keeping track of my appointments with the endocrinologist, the retinologist, and the orthopedic oncologist; making sure that I get test results sent to Dr. Nelson, and filling prescriptions as needed. (I could use a secretary…) But of course, I would not trade being home for anything, and also I realize that this part of the journey is kind of like growing up—it requires some new skills and tasks, but it is worth it. That's the trade-off of freedom versus responsibility (as I keep telling my teen-age sons).

I have met, in person and online, many post BMT patients who are in the throes of GVH to lesser and greater degrees than mine. I have been hobbling around on a cane, just about to feel sorry for myself, when I hear of someone who spent 40 days in the hospital with diarrhea, hooked up to feeding tubes and who knows what else. Then my bumpy road looks rather smooth…I take a big breath and quiet my whiny voices and try to just keep on keeping on.

The days and months go by, each with certain advances in my health and also with a few setbacks. It is with wonder that I look at all the healthy people walking around, oblivious to their cells or their blood counts or potassium levels or any of the ways their body is functioning. Healthy bliss, I guess. My vigilant awareness sometimes gets in the way of just getting through the day, but time will pass and that too will change, I am sure.

So why my "beautiful" leukemia? I have to admit, that phrase just popped into my head after about four days in the hospital and I was beginning to see that I was in for something Big. I didn't know what it meant. Now I think it is the fact that this near disaster took me and my family and a veritable community of people on an incredible journey. A journey that has not ended for me, although most of the guestbook writers have taken the caringbridge site off their "frequent list" and have gone back to their lives. Thank heavens for that. A few people still check up in the site regularly, like it's an old friend, and I post the various comings and goings. I seem to be out of the woods, as they say, and so we all move on. And that is beautiful! The whole thing that brought us together, and now drifts back into the lovely flow of life is, in my mind, beautiful.

And so in keeping with the idea that my experience might help somebody embarking on a similar journey, I humbly offer the following:

HOW TO BE A PATIENT
A few tips for anyone dealing with doctors, nurses and hospitals

1. As much as possible, be aware of what is happening to you, around you, and what's being said about you. If you can't be aware, maybe you're woozy from medication or just too scared to really listen, ask a friend or family member to be aware for you. A third party, a more rational listener, can be an essential part of your team. Doctors sometimes talk about their patients in the third person—right in front of the patient—especially if it is a teaching hospital and there is a team in attendance. That's all well and good and you should cooperate the best you can, but the bottom line is: it's your health, and in the case of serious illness, it's your life. So, open your eyes and ears and pay attention! Or get a friend to do so.

2. Having said that about being "aware", another side to that idea is deciding how much you want to know. There will be a lot of facts and figures thrown at you about your disease/condition. I learned, early on, that I did NOT want a lot of the statistics about my cancer; they were pretty dismal and not good for me to hear. I didn't want to

hear worst-case scenarios or the worst side effects of a medicine or treatment. I would tell the docs or nurses periodically, "That's enough. Don't need to hear that." Of course, there are those who want to know everything about their disease, want to know all the stats, and want to research it to the nth degree. That is another equally good way to cope—as long as you are consciously deciding your approach, not just letting the information blindside you.

3. Ask questions. If you don't understand what they're talking about, <u>ask</u>. If you didn't quite catch it the first time, <u>ask</u>. And <u>ask again</u>. Don't worry about being a pest— you have a right to know and to understand. My experience showed me that the doctors and nurses did not mind at all if I kept asking questions. They actually appreciated it and as a result I became more knowledgeable about my care.

4. Know this: The nurses are your best allies during your hospital stay. Every once in a while, if you are able, imagine yourself in their shoes. I would bet you come away from that thinking in amazement about what they do, how much they know. They are moving constantly, quietly and efficiently, drawing blood, setting up IVs, taking your "vitals", refreshing your water pitcher, recording data, dispensing meds—they do it all. Talk to them. Ask how <u>they're</u> doing, if they have families or pets or hobbies. And let them know how it goes with you. Use your manners and remember that you are not in a hotel getting room service. You're sick and you are part of a team—nurses, doctors, orderlies, all the people working in the hospital—all working together towards your health and recovery.

5. Write things down (or ask someone to write for you) such as medicines, any changes in meds, the name(s) of your condition or disease, and any procedures the doctor may be suggesting. You are in a world with its own language when you are in a hospital and it takes some getting used to. It's almost impossible to remember it all, so write it down.

6. If you're scared, tell your nurse. Tell your doctor. Even if you think you shouldn't be scared, tell them anyway. Let yourself be comforted. When you are admitted for a long stay, such as I was for leu-

kemia, you will probably have many of the same nurses in rotation. Let yourself trust the nurses. Give over to the fact that you need help, you're in a different world, and all your old defenses and coping mechanisms may not work so well in this new situation.

7. Pain management is of utmost importance. If you hurt, get relief. Tell someone, don't suffer in silence. Pain can actually hinder healing, as well as drag you down emotionally.

8. Whenever possible, have a sense of humor. I found myself in so many absurd situations—my pajamas becoming ridiculously big; the outfit I donned to walk in the halls; when driving my IV pole out in the hallway, I felt like I was in bumper cars…I could NOT get that thing to drive straight. These things were funny, and seeing them that way helped me as well as those who were taking care of me.

9. I highly recommend doing SOMETHING with your room— whether it's pictures of loved ones on the walls or a pretty quilt on your bed—anything to make the room yours for the duration of your stay. I can understand the rationale of not investing too much energy in "decorating"—it might seem like you're there to stay. Some people like to pretend they're not there (we call this "denial") and drown themselves in the television. But putting up some touches of your own in the hospital room has a dual purpose: it reassures you that you're still you (you have the pictures to prove it!) but it also lets the doctors and nurses know a bit about you too. The more they know— about your family, where you live, your interests—the more they can attend to you personally. Then you are not just any generic patient with a disease—you are a mother or a grandfather, you are a parachutist or gardener, a farmer or a chef. Pictures paint a thousand words and they can fill in the blanks for those dedicated people who are working so hard to make you well.

10. Ask for help. Let people help. These are not the same thing, but close. Unless you have been a mean curmudgeon all your life, you will have someone who wants to help you. (Even if you were such a curmudgeon, you may still have some to call on. My father was such an example—he became meaner and meaner as he inched in demen-

tia towards his death, but there were still people who cared and inquired after him). So if you need a foot rub, ask for it. If you need someone to call your sister and ask her to send more pajamas, ask. Asking for help is hard for almost everybody. Often friends, neighbors and family want to help but they don't know what to do. Give them a task. Ask for their help. Part two of this concept is then letting people help. Someone arrives in your room and offers to tidy up your papers and magazines, or wants to go and get the DVD cart, let them! In my first weeks in the hospital, I used to feel so powerless and useless when my friends would be buzzing around my room, bringing me fresh water, offering to wash a few things, straightening up my bedside table. I felt like I should jump up and help them. NO!! Let them help, I soon learned. They want to help. Heck, they want to cure you but since they can't, bringing a box of tissues is something.

11. And last but not least—be kind to yourself. Be easy on yourself, inside and out. Your amazing body is trying valiantly to recover. You may be slammed from chemo; nauseated and exhausted and wrung out. I know how that feels and there were times when I was angry that my body let me down. But when I could get quiet and focus on the inside of me, I was immensely cheered by the idea of all the cellular activity going on, so many chemical actions and reactions taking place all the time. My blood, my bones, my organs—all that amazingly beautiful stuff doing its silent work 24/7. We scarcely acknowledge it unless we're sick. So take a moment and love your cells and your body…be good to yourself. Get well.